A Better Life

A Better Life

How our darkest moments can be our greatest gift

CRAIG HAMILTON

with Will Swanton

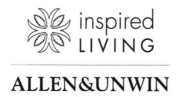

ALLEN&UNWIN

First published in Australia in 2012

Inspired Living, an imprint of
Allen & Unwin
Sydney, Melbourne, Auckland, London

83 Alexander Street
Crows Nest NSW 2065
Australia
Phone: (61 2) 8425 0100
Fax: (61 2) 9906 2218
Email: info@allenandunwin.com
Web: www.allenandunwin.com

Cataloguing-in-Publication details are available from the National Library of Australia
www.trove.nla.gov.au

ISBN 978 1 74237 973 9

Typeset in 12/16 pt Bembo by Midland Typesetters, Australia

10 9 8 7 6 5 4 3 2 1

For Louise, who did not lose faith in me when I almost lost faith in myself. Your love, guidance and support lifted me up and enabled me to see the light again.

Contents

'If you want to make God laugh, tell him your plans.'

Woody Allen

Foreword

Mental ill health in Australia has been increasingly recognised by ordinary Australians as the greatest contributor to human suffering, unfulfilled promise and loss of economic productivity among all of the health problems we face. Suicide kills more Australians under the age of 40 than any other cause, and the World Economic Forum reported in 2011 that mental illness now equals cardiovascular disease as the main threat to GDP growth in developed economies. And 35 per cent of Australians rate mental health among the top three issues confronting our nation in the 21st century. Only 10 per cent of Europeans and Americans possess this insight.

This is why Craig Hamilton deserves our respect and gratitude. He has been open, honest and courageous in his determination to tell his story, helping to sweep aside the tenacious clouds of silence, stigma and ignorance that have shrouded mental illness until recently. His personal qualities in the face of a hugely disturbing and life-threatening illness have enabled him to transcend his own ordeal, and achieve a rare level of wisdom and generosity through which he seeks to help others. His is a very moving and uplifting story, told with typical Novocastrian commonsense and compassion. He is a public figure and a respected journalist and this has increased the impact of his story. Many prominent sportspeople, politicians and artists have followed this path in recent years. Few, however, have been health professionals or come from the world of business and finance.

It takes real courage to be on the frontline, to be one of the first over the top. It still takes courage to disclose and share one's story of mental illness. Judgement and stigma still cause some people to turn away in fear and confusion. I am sure Craig looks forward, as do I, to the day when such responses become just as unacceptable as racism and sexism. That day is coming soon thanks, in part, to Craig and people like him.

The need for open discussion and disclosure of mental ill health in the same way we speak openly of our physical health challenges is one of the key messages Craig conveys through his writing and as a role model. Another is that mental illness, despite its complexity and potential severity, is eminently treatable. Not only is a normal life quite achievable, but so it is a special contribution.

Most of the misery and blight on lives resulting from mental illness is preventable with modern holistic treatment that often includes, but never solely relies upon, medication (even though for many people, including Craig, the latter is absolutely essential). Yet most people with mental illness have poor or belated access to care, and the quality and stability of this care lags way behind that found in mainstream healthcare. Mental illness receives only 7 per cent of the health budget, yet it creates 13 per cent of the health burden and, worse still, has greatest impact during young adulthood and the most productive years of life. The federal government has just begun to invest more heavily in mental healthcare and to back desperately overdue innovation and re-engineering of the system. However, most state governments (who remain responsible for the specialist mental health system) are really struggling to engage genuinely with this reform agenda. Craig gives examples of some of the financial and other barriers faced in obtaining state-of-the-art treatment. The only way we will overcome this neglect, which is costing lives and futures every day, is if Australians build on the awareness Craig has helped to create and demand that all of our political leaders and policy makers invest and innovate to ensure that all of us, not just the lucky ones, can expect the same quality in healthcare for mental illness as for physical illness.

Professor Patrick McGorry, AO, MD BS, PhD,
FRCP, FRANZCP
Australian of the Year 2010

Introduction

There are positives in the suffering? Gifts hidden in the pain?

Twelve years ago, my life unravelled with a manic explosion on Broadmeadow train station in Newcastle. I thought I was Jesus Christ incarnate ready to save all humankind. The psychosis followed a clinical depression that had engulfed me for most of the year. At my lowest point I experienced suicidal thoughts. I cannot claim to have embraced the notion of the whole shebang being any sort of blessing.

Now, however, I regard the year my world broke as a watershed in my life. Before Broadmeadow, my life was so terribly out of balance, in every area, that mental illness was nearly inevitable. I was taken to James Fletcher Psychiatric Hospital. Placed in lockdown. The diagnosis was delivered: bipolar 1 disorder—bipolar experienced with both mania and psychosis. (Bipolar 2 disorder has the same depressive symptoms but without full-blown mania or psychosis.) Life would never be the same again. I assumed it meant life would be worse.

Incredibly, despite all the bumps, bruises and scars inflicted, life's been better. The greatest challenges, adversities and hardships have sparked the most significant periods of personal growth. There have been countless positives in my twelve-year dance with mental illness.

Don't get me wrong—it's been traumatic, and the fight continues. Some of this I wouldn't wish on anyone's worst enemy. I've done all the soul searching: why me? Why anyone? What is the *meaning* of all this? The turning point came when I realised *I* had the power to change. My thoughts, decisions and actions used to go unchallenged. They were made without consideration for the consequences. If someone else suffered as a result of what I did or said, well, that wasn't my problem. I refused to take responsibility for outcomes unless, of course, they were favourable.

A life lived so recklessly and selfishly deserved to result in chaos. In the fallout, I needed to be honest about the way I was living. I could keep my life hectic, stressful and dysfunctional or go the opposite way and start listening to what my soul was really crying out for: peace, happiness, self-respect and the most powerful emotion of all, hope. Change was possible. It was possible!

I have survived, but so many others with a mental health issue are tempted to give up. I know it because I was there, too. I've written this book because I want them, and their family and friends, to know that there are people who understand—and the number is increasing as awareness is raised. You're depressed? I know how you feel. I've tumbled into pits of depression so severe that I never thought I would ever climb out. You're suicidal? I've been in the deepest, darkest, ugliest places you can imagine, but here's the moral to my story: I have clawed my way free. Which means you can, too.

Parramatta Stadium

4 SEPTEMBER 2010: Commentary duties for ABC Radio have taken me to Sydney's Parramatta Stadium. The bright lights of a cold September night. The Eels are playing the Warriors in the National Rugby League. Huge game. Massive atmosphere. Enough electricity to burn the joint to the ground. Adrenaline runs through every aisle, fills every seat, infiltrates everyone's bloodstream. This is high-voltage, elite sport—but I'm running on empty. The time bomb starts its march towards detonation. Tick-tock, tick-tock: seven hours to go.

'You OK, mate?'

My co-commentator, Steve Mortimer, knows my history with bipolar disorder. He knows my moods can swing clean off their hinges. So he asks me again.

'You OK?'

I felt fine driving to the game. Fine-ish walking up the steel spiral staircase to the media area. Steve and I hunker down in the ABC's commentary booth. I do my normal preparation: studying the program, checking off the players' names, matching the unfamiliar players to the numbers on their backs. Tick-tock. I'm behind the microphone for a studio air check. I still feel fine. I know the danger signs for a manic explosion and none of the flags have been raised—yet.

I tell Steve that I'm good to go. The game starts and we begin our call. I'm doing the live play-by-play commentary while Steve, one of league's finest players, a former NSW and Australia halfback, provides the expert analysis. Our broadcast is going to Queensland, NSW, the ACT and New Zealand. Hundreds of thousands of listeners are relying on us for accurate and informed details. The game is only fifteen minutes old when I realise I'm fading fast. I'm so flat, mugged by fatigue. This is a big game and an important call, but my words are hollow and insincere. I bluff my way through on counterfeit commentary.

The Eels are flogged. Their captain, Nathan Cayless, does a lap of honour for his 259th and final match. And Cayless's retirement is a big deal; one of those genuinely emotional sporting moments when a radio commentator is duty-bound to paint a precise and entertaining verbal picture for his listeners. But I'm so devoid of energy that I can barely string a sentence together. The exhaustion is overwhelming. I'm lucky to stay in my seat, low and getting lower, grinding to a halt at every level of mental and physical function. I feel like a plane falling from the sky. Steve keeps taking sideways glances. 'You sure you're OK?' Truth be told, all I really want to do is curl up under the desk and sleep until further notice. To hell with the Eels. To hell with Nathan Cayless. To hell in a hand-basket with the NRL. Afterwards, my mates will say they've never heard me so uninspired. They think it's because the Warriors' victory has booted my hometown team, the Newcastle Knights, out of the finals. They could not be more wrong. If only it were that simple.

I just don't care about anything. I don't care about the game, the result; nothing seems to matter. We're all wasting our time even being here; it's all so meaningless. The Parramatta faithful have come out in force to farewell their captain. I'm wholly uninterested. At halftime, a ten-minute break, I'd normally zip out to the media common room where journalists from print, radio and TV converge to chat, dissect the game and grab a bite to eat. But I avoid everyone tonight; the thought of a single conversation too much to bear. I'm holed up in the commentary booth like I'm hiding in a cave, door closed, speaking to no-one.

Tick-tock. I need space. 'You OK, mate?' I keep assuring Steve that I am. He starts hitting me with more questions: 'How's your family?', 'How's the health been lately?', 'You doing well with that?'

I say, 'Yes, yes, I've been great thanks, mate. Let's get on with it.' He looks at me with concern: I'll always remember the real concern on his face. Finally, it's pens down. Work is finished. Time to go to my temporary home. Steve shakes my hand, holding the grip a little longer than usual. He looks me in the eye and tells me to look after myself.

If I can, I will.

On the way out, I see two blokes I know pretty well. One is Steve Mascord, a sideline eye for the ABC and a respected writer on rugby league for newspapers and magazines. The other is Rod Reddy, the assistant coach at Parramatta and formerly a legendary player with St George Illawarra. I would normally say hello to both without a second thought but the stranger inside me puts his head down and walks straight past them without saying a single word. This is unbelievable to me: even as I'm striding past, I can't believe I'm ignoring them. I want to talk to them—but I can't. They must think I'm the rudest bloke on the planet but I just don't care. I leave Parramatta Stadium and head for the heart of Sydney. The night is but a pup.

1 The truth

Depression. Let me tell you about the real deal. Wrap every heartache and sadness of your life into a clenched fist of black cloud and that's what it feels like when the darkness moves in. Depression has been completely debilitating on every level of my being. There's been the total and utter lethargy; the extreme negative thoughts that have made me embrace the notion of the darkest possible night of the human soul—suicide. There really have been times when death has seemed like the only way out. It's just sheer suffering—that's the best way I can describe depression. It's a suffering so acute that, even though I've always tried to live life to the fullest, even though I *love* life, ending it has felt like the only way to ease the pain.

I have great empathy for people who try to take their own lives. I didn't want to but it just felt like the only reasonable option: the only route to *get away*. I can't think straight when I'm depressed. I can't eat. I can barely stand the thought of seeing another person, even those I adore. I don't want to drag everyone else down. I don't want to be a burden.

My wife, Louise, is a wonderful woman. We have three children I would take a bullet for: Josh, twenty; Amy, eighteen; and Laura, fourteen. But when I'm strangled by depression, there's just no respite and not even the thought of my family can snap me out of it. The cloud is just so thick that there is no sign of sunshine, anywhere. All I want to do is escape. I have to get away.

Thankfully, this state does not last forever. It is transient and I know it will pass. That's solace during these periods. If you have experienced severe depression, you already know what I'm talking about. It's a living hell: *I cannot get better, I cannot get better; I don't know why but I cannot get better.* It's not as if I have three or four hours of feeling poorly but then the rest of my day is manageable. The gloom is overwhelming and complete.

> **If you're depressed right now, you need help from anywhere you can get it.**

When I'm in deep, when the low is so all-consuming it feels like a knife is digging into the very core of my soul, the feeling lasts more than days or weeks. It goes on for *months*. My longest depression has hung around for nine months. It's torturous. I push and strain with all my might but the boulder refuses to shift. I know suicide would destroy my family and friends. I know it can impact on an entire community. But when a depression is in full swing, suicidal thoughts are as persistent as they are uninvited.

Why am I telling you this? Why don't I take these stories to my grave? Because I don't want to be silent. I want something good to come from my struggles. And if you're depressed right now, you need help from anywhere you can get it. Silence is cowardly and prevents the sharing of knowledge. Insufficient knowledge kills people, families and relationships. I am not prepared to sit on my hands and let that happen. I know how easily a mental illness can strike the unlikeliest suspects but most importantly of all, and here's the moral to the story, I know how it can be overcome. I know what's on the other side of every rough patch: good times, the natural highs of contentment and wellbeing—the best kinds of highs. In my experience, the good times outweigh the bad by ten to one. That's a good ratio. That's a full life. If I can help educate people about the realities of mental illness by sharing my knowledge, I will always endeavour to be truthful, even brutally so. If anyone out there is prepared to listen, I will always talk.

Abraham Lincoln said this nearly 200 years ago and it's as true now as it's ever been: 'The probability that we may fall in the struggle ought not to deter us from the support of a cause we believe to be just.' I think it's important to try to make a difference, big or small, noticed or unnoticed, successful or not. I want to increase understanding of mental illness. That's my lot in life. That's my mission statement. If there is one sentence in this book, one word that improves awareness or the quality of someone's life, I will have succeeded in spectacular fashion. I want my story to be thrown into the pot of knowledge. I want people to be armed with enough information to recognise traits, symptoms and behavioural patterns in those they're working with, sharing relationships with, raising families with; people they've grown up with, been friends with. I want to help them intervene before it's too late. Everything I have come to know about depression, mania, bipolar and chemical imbalances will be relayed in these pages.

'You must be the change you wish to see in the world.'
Gandhi

There is always the temptation to keep my travails private, put them in a vault for all time and make Louise promise to never tell a soul. Perhaps it would be better for my family if I concentrated solely on getting through another morning, another afternoon, another night. If I concentrated on no-one but myself. We've had a number of meetings, believe me, to thrash out whether this should remain a private or public crusade. We've decided, together, to tell the truth, and hope we can make a positive contribution to the debate. I feel no embarrassment whatsoever. Louise has misgivings, of course. She's very protective of the kids and so am I. They're the number one consideration, but they're old enough to understand the issue now and they've given me their consent.

They were babies when I was diagnosed. Now they're teenagers. They've grown up with me being like this. They haven't vetoed any part of my journey and I thank them wholeheartedly for that. Louise went through the manuscript and sections of it definitely made her emotional. She shed a tear while putting together her own chapter. However, it should be noted that she still cries at the end of *An Officer and a Gentlemen* and *Pretty Woman*.

There are bad memories in here that I'm sure she would rather forget instead of having me tell the world. This is serious stuff. I know I'm not exactly the textbook husband; I'm not even the same man she married. Louise didn't grow up hoping she would find a handsome prince who would end up in a psychiatric hospital with a lifelong affliction. But Louise knows what I'm trying to do here, even if it makes her roll her eyes. She supports me 100 per cent. Well, 99 per cent: she worries that publishing a book will lead to another episode; she frets about me being more concerned with everyone else's welfare than my own. But you wouldn't be reading any of this without her selfless consent, either. A weight has been lifted from my shoulders by telling the truth. Opening up is the ultimate liberation.

I am a better husband with bipolar disorder than I was without. I am a better man. People say the bravest thing I ever did was go public. To do speaking engagements to rooms full of strangers, to write books, to be an ambassador for *beyondblue*, to talk about mental health on the radio. I disagree. The bravest thing I ever did—the bravest thing I am still doing—is living through it in the first place. The talking part is easy. I'm telling the truth, so what's there to be worried about? Hiding would be harder. I say 'I'm living through it' in the present tense because this is an ongoing and never-ending battle. Every day is somewhere between a challenge and the fight of my life. It's taken me twelve years to feel that my plan of attack is right. Hopefully I can help you avoid it taking so long!

Stuff the stigma: mental illness must be confronted instead of whispered about. There should be no shame in it. Thankfully, the stigma is fading: organisations such as *beyondblue*, SANE Australia and the Black Dog Institute in Sydney do tremendous work. High-profile people such as Andrew Johns and Wally Lewis have made an enormous difference by revealing their own battles—but there's still a way to go. The lack of understanding lingers.

> Mental illness must be confronted instead of whispered about.

There's still a desire to sweep it away like a dirty secret and I'm not prepared to let that happen. I understand the unease because I used to feel it myself. I never wanted to know about any of this either, mental illness was creepy and dangerous—until it was forced upon me. Pre-bipolar, when compassion was not exactly an emotion I was overly familiar with, if someone told me they were depressed, I told them to get over themselves and man up. Stop being such a bloody sook. How wrong I was, how naive and stupid.

Perhaps I was so ignorant and uncaring that actually getting bipolar disorder was the only way to have some sense knocked into me. If that's the case, I've been given my comeuppance. I have learned my lesson, good and proper. I have been shown in no uncertain terms that physically, emotionally and spiritually, clinical depression is possibly the most painful experience a human being can have—but I've also learned it is temporary.

In the twelfth century BC, Persian poets wrote about a king who asked his men to create a ring that would make him happy when he was sad, and sad when he was happy, to remind him of the temporary nature of all emotions. The sages handed him a ring with the following words written on it: 'This too will pass.' Those with a mental illness can do more than persevere. We can prosper. Depression, too, will pass. I must have repeated that to myself a million times. This too will pass.

Lift-off

There's more to tell about the night of Parramatta Stadium. But first I want to fill you in on how I got to this point: It was the year 2000 when the first big bang came. I was about to catch the XPT to Sydney to cover the Olympic Games for the ABC. One step off the platform at Broadmeadow train station and I would have been on my way. A dream would have come true.

For a sports reporter, nothing tops an Olympics—nothing. The high point of my working life would arrive when the train departed. It was all ready to go, lined up on Platform 1, inclining towards Sydney like a silver bullet. I'd escaped the coalmines, made a rapid rise through the media ranks, been employed by the most prestigious broadcaster in the land. Now the greatest sports event in the world was at my fingertips. The epicentre of the athletic universe was a two-hour trip away. But just as I was about to board, just as I was saying goodbye to Louise and some mates, I had the manic explosion to top them all.

I believed with all my heart and soul that I was Jesus Christ incarnate. I wasn't going to Sydney to cover the Olympics for the ABC: I had no doubt in my mind that I, Jesus Christ, was scheduled to take the podium at the closing ceremony with Nelson Mandela. We would deliver a message of such love, hope and goodwill that all mankind would be rescued. Together, Nelson and I would eradicate war, hatred, anger, discrimination. I believed this wholeheartedly. Jesus Christ incarnate, however, never made it to the Olympics.

He didn't even get a seat on the XPT. He abused a very close friend. Fuck off! Don't you know we're all dead? Don't you see? The Son of God lashed out at police like a wild animal before an army of men in blue could restrain him. I suffered the indignity of being thrown in the back of a paddy wagon in the heart of my hometown. I was taken to James Fletcher Hospital and spent eleven days in a psychiatric ward. I wasn't in possession of divine powers bestowed upon me by the good Lord. To my eternal surprise, I wasn't the Son of God at all. I was Craig Hamilton, I had bipolar 1 disorder and life would never be the same again.

2 Blessings from the fallout

There *had* to be a consequence for living the way I did. You can't exist with my kind of innate restlessness without a collapse. I used to look for answers to my anxieties in all the wrong places: material possessions, career achievements, the opinions of others. I was barking up three wrong trees. My diagnosis was not the start of a slide into oblivion; rather, it was the start of everything coming good.

Without a word of a lie, hand on heart, despite the road I'm travelling on having potholes the size of the outback, I am happier with bipolar than I was without it. I'm a more complete human being. I'm a more understanding and compassionate human being. Initially, undoubtedly, being diagnosed with mental illness made me think I'd been dealt a dud hand, but I'm here to tell you that ace–king isn't the only way to win a game of 21. There will be no descent into sentimentality here, but I can honestly say that outside marrying Louise and the three miracles of Josh, Laura and Amy, mental illness is the greatest thing that has ever happened to me.

> My diagnosis was not the start of a slide into oblivion; rather, it was the start of everything coming good.

It's forged layers of self-awareness I would never have experienced otherwise. Introspection is now performed with an attention to detail previously reserved for analyses of the outside world. Not that it's all plain sailing. Shortly before getting started on this book, despite more than a decade of self-maintenance and knowledge-gathering, I was still swallowed by depression.

Only through expert and heartfelt care, a tweaking of my prescribed medicines and—another shock, horror—the influence of alternative therapies I used to dismiss as hocus-pocus, did I return to balance. That three-month swirling cloud of depression is still fresh in my mind, but I feel stronger for having survived another storm, and I've since gone more than a year feeling better than I ever have.

> 'There are two great days in a person's life—the day we are born and the day we discover why.'
> William Barclay

Every fight toughens me up, gives me another layer of insight into the enemy, adds to my own bulging files of information. I've done more than 300 public presentations on the topic of mental health in the last six years, all of them relating to the hardships I've encountered but also, importantly, to the triumphs. These public engagements have been the most rewarding work experiences of my life. Don't get me wrong, I love ABC Radio. I feel privileged to be working for it and the support from the organisation has been unstinting when it comes to my mental health advocacy. But my public speaking comes from my heart. I've spoken in every state except Western Australia. I've been to Darwin, Cairns, Townsville and Brisbane. I've been to little places like Cloncurry and Muttaburra in Queensland and Condobolin in central NSW; from big cities to small communities hit by serious psychological problems. Rural life is tough and unforgiving and whole livelihoods can hang on something as fickle as the weather.

Depression is skyrocketing. There are droughts in some areas, floods in others. The tales are harrowing once you seek them out. Stress and worry are sticks of dynamite to mental illnesses that otherwise might never emerge in a lifetime. In every town, I tell my story as faithfully and truthfully as I can, take questions and afterwards talk to anyone who's up for a chat. The depth and breadth of mental health issues is as vast and diverse as the country itself. Hopefully it's good for people to hear my tale. I know it's good for me. When I've been down in the dumps or depressed myself, I've found that concentrating on someone else's woes has been a fantastic tonic. I'm trying hard to replace selfishness with selflessness. Helping: it's just terrific therapy. I end up forgetting what was bothering me in the first place.

The ripple effect is what I cherish: when a knowledgeable word touches someone I wouldn't have expected to be touched, or didn't even know existed. I give my spiel in a public forum, relate my own experiences, make sure everyone understands I'm ashamed of none of it, throw in my twenty cents worth and see where the ripples wash up. One day when I was talking about depression on Newcastle radio, a guy rang the studio and said, 'I feel like you're talking about me. I've had all those symptoms for the last three years. I've been suicidal four or five times.' I told him to hold the line so I could talk to him after the show. I wanted to help him; I wanted to know more. He'd made a big step just by picking up the phone.

Talking to him off air would have been perfect. But he said no, he couldn't do it—and hung up. That was terrible, hearing the line go dead. I felt ill. The following night, I had another speaking engagement in Newcastle. Afterwards, a girl of about fifteen or sixteen came up to the stage. She'd been crying and said she wanted to say thanks: the man who called the radio station the night before was her father. That's the ripple effect. That's why I will keep grabbing as many microphones as I can get my hands on.

3 Daring to open up

My first public talk was at a local school. *Will you come? We've got some kids here with depression. Can you help?* That's how it began. Very basic. I spoke for twenty minutes to a class of thirty kids. It went well and an invitation arrived to speak at a Catholic high school. That was a step up. I expected a much tougher crowd, given the ages of the students to be herded into the hall: Years 9, 10 and 11, mid-teens, not always the most attentive lot when a stranger is talking about this kind of issue. They gave me their full attention. The moment I saw the fascination on their faces I was shocked. They sat and listened to every single word. It was almost eerily quiet. That's when I realised I was on to something important. When someone like me can stand in front of a Year 11 class and they're not clockwatching or staring at their feet or sniggering and mucking up; when I could actually engage them and see the recognition in their eyes, I knew something significant was happening. I was thrilled my talk had gone down so well. At the very least, I liked the thought that some of these kids would leave the hall with more information than they had when they arrived.

But then a couple of them approached me—privately, a bit tentatively—when all their friends had left, to say their mum or

dad was depressed and they wanted advice on how to help. The
irony was obvious: they were in school, in the very place that
should be teaching them life skills, but until then they had known
nothing about such a large and real issue. Generations of Australians have entered adulthood clueless about it.

I'm glad to report that's changing. Openness is crucial. The
bigger the support network, the better for all of us. I am hopeless
at many things, believe me. Changing a light bulb is the upper
limit of my practical prowess. I have broken more things at home
than I have fixed, but I do know how to communicate. I know
what I'm talking about when I get up and take the microphone
on this subject. When someone tells me they're depressed, I know
exactly how they feel. You've been suicidal? Me too. You're losing
hope? Don't!

Writing this, I have nothing but positive thoughts. Perhaps this
is therapy for me, too: 'The best way to become acquainted with
a subject is to write a book about it,' says Benjamin Disraeli. The
dark times are only mentioned to contrast the brightness on the
other side. I can see the relief on the faces of the people I talk
to; the relief that someone knows where they're coming from.
Old or young, rich or poor—depression can hit anyone. I act
normally. I talk normally. I *am* normal. And if I can get through
depression, you can too. I can see the shame and embarrassment
washing off people when they realise they're not the only ones.
There should be no shame attached to any of this, except perhaps
among those who turn their backs on it.

You've been suicidal? Me too. You're losing hope?
Don't!

A group of financial advisers are having a conference. There is
an increasing level of anxiety and depression in their ranks. I tell
them how my life unravelled at Broadmeadow, how my blow-up

has changed my priorities, how I'm so much better off because of it. I emphasise the importance of work–life balance: getting off your email when you can, turning off your phone, putting your BlackBerry away. (Don't get me started on social media! I have the strongest views that I'll ram down your throat soon enough.)

When I'm finished talking, one guy comes up and says, 'Mate, that's alright for you. When you're not working, no-one needs to contact you. I'm a team leader. I've got to have my phone on 24 hours a day, seven days a week.' I tell him no-one needs their phone on 24/7—I doubt the prime minister does. But he's adamant: he reckons he's so important that his clients need to be able to contact him at any time of the day or night. I tell him, well, if that's the case, you must be indispensable. And then I tell him that cemeteries all over Australia are full of indispensable people just like him. He turns on his heel, walks away. He isn't angry or offended, he just takes it on the chin and leaves me standing there.

About two months later, the same guy sends me an email. It says thanks for the message. His wife has been trying to tell him the same thing for years: make more time with the kids, spend more time with her, have a life outside work, find a way for them to go hand-in-hand. She's wanted him to *relax,* but he just hasn't been listening. Another ripple effect.

> Anyone can improve their mental health as effectively as we can better our physical fitness. The key is making a conscious decision to do it.

One of the mysteries of the human psyche: why do we so often fail to listen to the people who care about us the most, who know us the best—sometimes better than we know ourselves? Why does familiarity makes us less inclined to heed their advice?

I believe as long as the message gets across, it doesn't matter where it originated. I'm glad I pricked that man's conscience. I'll gladly point out the consequences of ignoring problems because I can show him the scars from the fallout. I don't expect anyone, in any of my audiences, to have life-changing revelations right there and then. But if I chip away, give them something to take home and think about when their head hits the pillow, then mission accomplished. Anyone can improve their mental health as effectively as we can better our physical fitness. The key is making a conscious decision to do it.

Even a mentally healthy person can make their mind healthier. We're all on the same search. It's the nature of the human beast to seek happiness, but we have to admit some of our attempts are hopelessly misguided. The bigger house, the flash car: the further we get from those goals, the angrier and more frustrated we get, but deep down we know they're not the answer anyway. It's all in our heads. Inner turmoil needs inner answers. I didn't accept that and then came my meltdown at Broadmeadow. My journey since has been broken into two stages. For the first six years, I think I was on my L plates when it came to mental illness. Now I'm on my Ps. I look forward to becoming fully qualified some day.

I've certainly been around the block a few times. The stories I hear are raw, real and make me duty-bound to share my own stories because others do me the same honour. I was in Booleroo, near Port Pirie in South Australia, for a community forum of about 300 people. Two retired wheat farmers, aged in their 70s or 80s, were sitting down the front, having a fine old time, cracking jokes; a couple of good blokes enjoying each other's company. I imagine they had seen plenty of prosperous times on the land but by the weatherbeaten look of them, just as many rough times.

One of them approached me at the end of the night. He was no longer having a fine old time. White as a ghost, he shook my hand and thanked me for talking about a topic close to his heart. The suicide of his daughter had been haunting him for decades. It made a little more sense to him now.

One of the great poems I've read was written by my good mate Murray Hartin. Murray is a larger-than-life character well known throughout many bush towns in Australia for his unique brand of humour and excellent bush poetry. He wrote 'Rain from Nowhere' a few years ago—it's a very powerful poem and cuts straight to the heart of depression in farming communities across the country during the too-frequent periods of drought. That poem, I'm sure, has saved lives. Life is tough. So what? We all have obstacles to overcome. They're a pain in the neck. Big deal. Inspiration is everywhere.

As a child, Dr John Demartini, who featured in the documentary *The Secret*, had callipers on his legs and learning problems. He was helpfully informed from an early age that he would never amount to anything worthwhile. He would never be able to read or write. Dr Demartini was told this so often that he bought into the idea—until he was seventeen, when he met a man of insight and optimism, who told him he was a genius. Even if the full extent of his brilliance was yet to reveal itself, it was there nonetheless.

There's danger in letting other people define you.

All it took was the belief of one person to change his thinking. Dr Demartini now travels the world as a master motivator to millions of people. Not bad for a kid who was supposed to be illiterate and dull. There's danger in letting other people define you. I hate thinking about teenagers who are told they're a waste of space and then take those negative self-images into adulthood. The ramifications can be dire. Those teens have depression and self-destruction written all over them.

Dr Demartini says we *know* there will be ups and downs in life, so let's get through the lows and celebrate the highs. But be balanced in the way you perceive the successes and failures. People will always try to drag you down, but Dr Demartini says this: ignore them. A few bumps along the way: that's the way I like it. The alternative seems boring. The fantastic challenge is to keep learning and improving.

Anyone can be our teacher. We can pick up on admirable traits in others and adopt them ourselves. I've learned a great deal from my own family. They've shown me what unconditional love is all about. How it can rub off on others. How forgiveness can heal and how faith is the beginning of finding true meaning and worth. I intend to repay their gift to me in as many ways as possible. I used to take my family for granted, but that will never happen again.

When I get my own life in order, when I'm living what I consider to be my best life, everything else comes good around it. If I hold up my end of the bargain, the reward is having every-thing else fall into place—mind, body and soul. I just want to live right, all because I've made the conscious decision to improve myself.

The following is said to be written on the tomb of a bishop in the crypts of Westminster Abbey:

When I was young and free and my imagination had no limits, I dreamed of changing the world. As I grew older and wiser, I discovered the world not changed, so I shortened my sights somewhat and decided to change only my country. But it, too, seemed immovable. As I grew into my twilight years, in one last desperate attempt, I settled for changing only my family, those closest to me, but alas, they would have none of it. And now, as I lie on my deathbed, I suddenly realise: If only I had changed myself first, then by example I would have changed my family. From their inspiration and encouragement, I would have been able to better my country and, who knows, I might have even changed the world.

When you just can't sleep

4 SEPTEMBER 2010, evening:When you don't recognise the warning signs, you don't get the help you need. It's 10.30 p.m. I have to spend tonight in an inner-city Sydney hotel before catching an 8 a.m. flight to Canberra to cover another NRL game.The drive to town has been a blessing: traffic everywhere, all the cars and people and buildings and neon signs of the city like a living organism swaying back and forth, forcing me to focus. I check into my hotel. I am still dog-tired. I want to get to my room, turn out the light and sleep like the dead. I've stayed in this hotel so often that I know the staff, but tonight they look like faceless strangers. I still have no interest in human interaction and get my key while barely making a peep. Tick-tock. I crawl to my room, tiredness crushing me. I'm tempted to sleep on the floor before I even get to the bed. My brain is full of dull nothing, the calm before the psychotic storm.

I do not want to be here.

I want to be in Newcastle with Louise and the kids.

I want their familiarity.

I need their familiarity, some semblance of reassurance that it's not happening again. Is it happening again? I take my medication, 1000 milligrams of the mood-stabilising drug Epilim. Given how I've been feeling, I should fall asleep as soon as my head hits the pillow, but I'm lying on my back, brain short circuiting—and my eyes fly wide open.

The first flag is raised. I'm staring at the ceiling, ramping up. It's 12.30 a.m. . . . Here comes mania . . . 1.30 a.m. . . . Here's Johnny . . . 2.30 a.m. . . . my mind is revving like a V8 engine. I have to get to sleep but it's become impossible. Now I never want to sleep again. I've had bipolar disorder for more than a decade. I know what I need.

Managing stress levels, maintaining regular sleep patterns, taking my medications—they're all important. But near the top of the list is this: I must sleep all night, every night. If I don't, there will be trouble. Here comes trouble. My mood has done a complete U-turn. I'm wide awake, more awake than I've ever been in my life. I jump out of bed. Epilim is a mood stabiliser for depression or mania, whichever of the twin muggers gets me first. I've been waiting and waiting for the drug to kick in, waiting for the antidote to the snake's poison to take effect, foot tapping, uncontrolled and unwell.

Delusional thoughts start ricocheting off the walls. Hours pass like seconds. In the blink of an eye it's 3.30 a.m. My pupils are bulging like the kid's in A Clockwork Orange. *I'm wired. I walk to the window of my room and stare down at the streets of the swarming concrete jungle. Psychosis hits. I am no longer Craig Hamilton. I am St Francis of Assisi and I'm on a mission.*

4 The manila folder

Every step in the journey I'm learning new things about myself and the world. If we want life to be better, we need to keep growing, even when it gets a bit painful. I have a brown manila folder. Inside my brown manila folder are hundreds of letters and email printouts sent to me since I published my first book, *Broken Open*, in 2005. They are from people whose lives have been affected, directly or indirectly, temporarily or permanently, by bipolar disorder, depression, or any of the variations of mental illness that can take hold of anyone from a high school student to a high court judge.

Every piece of correspondence moves me. A young woman's mother has started treating her differently because her erratic behaviour can finally be explained. Another twenty-something woman takes the time to write from her hospital bed. She's been filled with renewed hope just when she was about to fall too low to recover.

It's a prized possession, my brown manila folder, because if I start doubting what I'm trying to do, when I wonder if anybody is listening, all these dog-eared bits of paper are a source of profound encouragement. It's filled with bravery because for many of the people who've contacted me, it's the first time they've told anyone their story. I'm honoured they've decided to tell me. Some go into great detail, others simply say thank you for helping me feel less alone. There's no long-lasting correspondence. We wish each other well and get on with it. We have to do most of the fighting on our own.

> 'A hero is one who knows how to hang on one minute longer.'
>
> Novalis

Some of the writers have had bipolar disorder for more than 30 years. Some are reeling from only recently finding out. Others are undiagnosed but can see the symptoms. (I get overwhelmed by the thought of how many people are battling undiagnosed demons. If you think there's a problem, see a doctor. Either way, you will have peace of mind.)

The things people go through. Everything from lying in job interviews about the lapses in employment records to trying to get their parents to understand how genuine the fight is. There's every trial and tribulation, from relationship breakdowns to losses of jobs and careers. Hospitalisations, bad experiences with medications, lost friendships. Difficult topics are addressed but the overriding theme of the brown manila folder is the most powerful one of all. *Hope.*

More than 70 per cent of the correspondence is handwritten, which makes it even more personal, as if people's lives and innermost thoughts have flowed from their veins, through their pens and onto the pages. Sometimes the letters are just a few lines. Sometimes they're three or four pages long.

One man from Western Australia started his email so simply: 'I'm just writing to let you know that because of your honesty, my two boys still have their father.' That man fills me with strength. If you think mental health issues are a figment of people's imaginations, read on. This is what's happening in the real world.

Here's another of these heartwarming gems:

I don't know how to begin this—so I'm just going to start. I'm twenty-three. In April I went backpacking for four months—what an adventure. I met a wonderful man and fell madly in love. I came home to Australia and my life fell apart. My relationship with my alcoholic mother hadn't changed—I didn't fit in with my friends any more and the job I went back to was running me into the ground. I went to my local GP who put me back on some antidepressants. Unfortunately they weren't working. I was such a mess.

My birthday was a terribly wet and miserable day. I was driving my mum to the airport when I got a flat tyre—my mobile phone didn't work and my mother was hailing a taxi—from there my day went downhill. Everyone (except my mum) forgot my birthday and I sat at home that night, confused. I called [the crisis helpline] Lifeline, not because I was suicidal but because I just wanted to tell someone how bad my day had been.

I picked myself up and carried on with my hectic schedule and pretended to the outside world that everything was fine. I'm the one that everyone comes to with their problems—yet when I needed someone, no-one was there. I hit a brick wall on a Wednesday night and saw my GP, who decided that I was to be admitted to hospital.

My mother was relieved as she would not have to deal with me any more. I called my boyfriend and told him what was happening—he was shocked but relieved I would be getting help. My aunt called to check on my progress and was horrified that I was going into hospital. 'Just snap out of it, you silly girl!' That night, like every other night, I did not sleep very well. I packed my clothes and your book that I started to read but did not have time to finish as life was too busy.

Once I was in these walls I felt like I could finally be me. I cannot tell you how many boxes of tissues I went through or Tim Tams were eaten in my first week. I finished your book and it made me realise that I needed to look after myself physically and mentally. The sad part is, I don't have a fantastic support system—so I'm relying on myself to get through this. People's reactions to me being in here have been fascinating—actually, devastating is the appropriate word for this.

Thankfully your book has kept me company and motivated me to work things out. I have a very long and lonely road ahead of me—but you have given me hope, hope that there is light at the end of this black tunnel. I'm still in hospital and will be for a few more weeks. I guess I just wanted to say thank you for sharing your story with me and thank you for the hope you have given me.

So what can we learn from this letter? My heart goes out to anyone trying to get through this alone. I greatly admire their resilience. I don't know if I would have survived by myself. For people who have been hospitalised, who are seriously ill but whose family has abandoned them, putting them in the too-hard basket without realising the gravity of the illness, all I can do is urge you to seek support from anyone you can. Just one person can make the difference; one person you feel understands. My heart really does go out to the lone wolves.

'Illness' is an interesting word. Some people don't like it. But bipolar is what it is: an illness—maybe it's even a disease, I don't know. Bipolar disorder speaks for itself: it's a disorder, but at different stages of my journey, all three of those terms have felt apt. An imbalance sounds right because of the dramatic mood shifts. Illness, disease—some terms sound harsher than others but I go through times when each of them feels absolutely appropriate. They're serious terms for a serious affliction.

5 Meeting David Mackenzie

When you're in the wars it's easy to assume you're the only person in the world who is facing serious challenges. When the pain kicks in it's tempting to think you're hard done by, or that life's punishing you for things you should've done, did do, or wanted to do. The thing is, life is complex—there are days that are good, days that are bad or nearly impossible, and days that are indifferent. What I've learned is that how you choose to experience life is up to you.

David Mackenzie might well have taught me more than anyone and it only took him 45 minutes. Meeting this incredible man was an honour; just an amazing and profound experience. I think everyone we meet can add a little to our lives, whether we realise it or not. Every conversation and connection helps us to keep moving forward. I only knew David for a brief while before he died but he will never be forgotten. 'Heroic' barely does him justice.

I first heard of David through colleagues who had interviewed him for ABC Radio in Newcastle. He was diagnosed with motor neurone disease when he was in his early 40s. One day he was fit and well, playing cricket, running between wickets in a game. He felt weakness in his legs and started feeling unwell. These were the first minor signs of something cruelly major. Within a week, maybe ten days, he was diagnosed with this incurable illness.

The illness had progressed quite a bit by the time I got to meet him. He was in his twilight by then, having already written one heartrending book, *Coming to Life*, which told the story of his death sentence of a diagnosis and how his spirituality helped him see silver linings. He had incredible faith which only built after his diagnosis. I would have expected it to be diminished: how could God do this to him and his family? They were good people, amazing people, incredible people—how could they deserve this?

If someone had to be given motor neurone disease, why not a murderer? Why not a sinner—someone who perhaps deserved a little punishment? Why David Mackenzie? The more his physical body deteriorated, the more his spiritual growth was building and strengthening. He believed it didn't matter what happened to his body because his spirit was heading to a better place. He had an increased understanding of his flesh being temporary, his spirit would go on. He was an incredible individual.

I arrived at his house and looked at the physical man. He was in a wheelchair. Basically he had no use of his limbs at all. He could *barely* move his arms or legs an inch. He could only operate his wheelchair with his chin or one of those devices like a straw. He'd blow into it to manoeuvre the chair. I got out my my tape recorder and a microphone and began the interview.

His speech was a bit shaky but he still had a spark. It was coming from inside him and his collapsed body couldn't contain it. His bristling energy was tangible. He just did not feel at all sorry for himself. I was thinking, Man, and I reckon I have it tough? I could walk out his door, get in my car, drive home, take a swim, go to a movie—anything I wanted. He was stuck. There's medication for what I have. This man had no cure. He was going to die sooner rather than later, and he knew it. I thought I had all these unfair worries and troubles and problems, but here was a guy who really did have an insurmountable hurdle . . . and he was counting his blessings? It shook me up.

He just had a very cheery outlook on life. I didn't know if I should laugh or cry. Even the title of his book, *Coming to Life*, had me looking twice. Coming *to* life? You serious? There's a typo in your title: you're dying! Yet again, I thought wrong. David's physical life was being taken from him, but who said that was the end of his existence? He did not see it that way and who could argue with him? His viewpoint was the only one that counted. What a wonderful outlook for someone whose days were numbered. It wasn't until I got to meet him, and also when I read his second book, *This Terminal Life* (which I was privileged enough to write the foreword to), that I properly understood his thinking.

> 'When I was five years old, my mother always told me that happiness was the key to life. When I went to school, they asked me what I wanted to be when I grew up. I wrote down "happy". They told me I didn't understand the assignment, and I told them they didn't understand life.'
>
> John Lennon

We all walk the path from life to death. It's the one certainty that every last one of us has in common: we are born and we are going to die, whether we like it or not. No amount of money, title or prestige can spare us that. The world's richest man is in for the same final fate as the poorest. That's the physical life. Afterwards, though, what then? David believed that was when the real fun and games were going to begin. He accepted his physical life was going to finish sooner than he expected or hoped for but in the big picture, although it was being hurried up, nothing had changed too much. He was always going to die, the only question had been when. Perhaps he was better off knowing. He could leave on his own terms. Nothing would be left unsaid—and he would join his family when they too passed away in their own good time.

David surrendered to that, believed in it. I want to surrender to it, too, while I'm still alive. I'm in no immediate danger of falling off the perch—or am I? It will happen one day, so I'd better make the most of whatever time I do have. It's such an obvious message, such a clear one, but one I never quite grasped before meeting David. He made the utmost of the short time he had remaining. He wrote two wonderful books of strength and hope. He wrote personal messages in those books to his children and grandchildren that they will have all their lives. It was time and energy well spent.

I met his wife and kids. Beyond amazing. The physical and emotional support they provided him, while they grappled with their own sadness about his diagnosis, was constant, incredible and infinite. It was a privilege to be allowed into their home, to see them in their own environment. They were so warm and welcoming after I'd been so apprehensive walking up the steps to their front door. I really didn't know what to expect. I'd never met anyone with motor neurone disease and certainly didn't have much knowledge of the illness, other than the fact that there was no cure and that it ravaged the body. But once I got over the initial feeling of 'Gee, this guy is terribly handicapped', I felt very comfortable in his presence—because he made me so.

There was a cheeky grin on his face, as if he knew something we didn't. He was able to laugh at his situation. How wonderful is that? He put me very much at ease. Another lesson learned: how I treat other people will have a marked and lasting effect on how they treat their own circle. As my old mate Nelson Mandela says: 'And as we let our own light shine, we unconsciously give other people permission to do the same.'

David knew other people might feel uncomfortable in his presence so he used humour to break the ice. His strength of character and acceptance of his illness made it so much easier for his family. If he was sitting around in misery, if it was all doom and gloom, if he spent all day and night crying 'Why me? Why me?' that would have rubbed off just as much as the bravery. It wasn't all upside, of course. David experienced depressions. He wrote about wanting his life to be over, too. I'm sure he had some terribly dark and challenging nights.

I received an email from his brother when David passed away. I remember sitting at my desk, numb. It was sobering to realise he really had gone. David was such a huge spirit that it was tempting to think not even motor neurone disease could stop him. But he was gone. He was a bloke who made a huge difference with his inspiring, positive outlook on life.

> David taught me that no matter what confronts me,
> I have to look it in the eye.

David taught me to get the best possible result from whatever situation I was in. He taught me that no matter what confronts me, I have to wrestle with it, take it on. I have to realise that I'm stronger than I think and that when a fight is on, I can hold my own. I realise that I didn't get to see every facet of David Mackenzie in our 45-minute chat. That unless I actually lived his experience, 24 hours a day, seven days a week, I could never get the warts-and-all-story. But the picture I was presented with was never to be forgotten. If David Mackenzie wasn't a hero, no-one is.

After dark

5 SEPTEMBER 2010, 3.30 a.m.: *Let's face it, suffering is uncomfortable. It takes us to the edge. Sin City throbs with the drunks, the drug addicts, the lovers, the fighters, the hopeless, the depraved—and, soon enough, me. St Francis of Assisi knows suffering when he sees it. I must leave my hotel room and save these mortal souls. I will walk the streets and perform miracles. They. Will. All. Be. Saved.*

I have a heightened, almost supernatural, feeling of connectedness to all other human beings. I am invincible, immune to negativity, flying on a higher and more enlightened plane. I will show the beaming light to all those in my path. It is complete sensory overload. The flight of ideas. They're fleeting yet grandiose.

I am St Francis of Assisi. Of course I am! It is so clear to me, so rational. I must rescue the poor and the homeless. There is no time to waste. I can feel the suffering on the streets, I can smell it. The empathy is extreme. I want to give these people my heart. I fling open the door of my hotel room, striding down the corridor, sweeping through the foyer like any religious figure worth his robes.

Staff have bemused looks on their faces. Pointing and grinning, they think I've had too many drinks, that I got stuck into the minibar after the footy. They think I'm pissed as ten parrots. Now I'm on George Street, in the very heart of Sydney, well past the witching hour. It's 3.30 a.m.

Nothing good happens after midnight. St Francis of Assisi is wearing a T-shirt—and nothing else. From the waist down, walking along the busiest street in the busiest city in Australia, I am naked.

6 Awakening

I am not a religious person, which makes me wonder why, when catapulted into mania, I develop such a strong religious bent. I used to live in a complete spiritual vacuum. I worked all week, played sport and had a few beers, repeating the same old routine for years on end. That kind of existence seems extraordinarily shallow to me now. Then, I would dismiss anything remotely spiritual as mumbo jumbo rolled into gobbledegook sprouted by zealots—I had no connection to any of it. I rarely attended church while growing up and I still don't, unless someone is getting married, christened or buried.

I was kicked out of class at Sunday school for talking and failing to pay attention. These days, however, a disinclination to get suited up and attend church every Sunday morning has not precluded me from experiencing an awakening that has become the most stunning part of my journey. I have come to accept the possibility of deeper levels of existence.

Being a former coalminer, I'm a bit uncomfortable calling it a 'spiritual awakening', but I'm very comfortable calling it 'an awakening of a spiritual nature'. Am I hedging my bets? Probably! All I know is that I've been blown apart in ideals and beliefs; in mind, body and soul. Until recently, nothing much had changed since Sunday school. I was still failing to pay attention, still talking too much in class. It was overcompensation for my fear of the unknown. Now the unknown is what I want to embrace. We live and learn, or at least we attempt to. Some of us take longer than others.

> 'Knowing yourself is the beginning of all wisdom.'
> Aristotle

Can you have an awakening without fully understanding what that awakening is? Yep, because I'm having it. A previously unreal world of spirituality is starting to feel pretty real. The beauty of a more spiritual path is that no-one else can control what inspires me or what I decide is rubbish. I'm the sole judge and jury of my own beliefs. I know what lifts my spirits and rings true and I know what doesn't.

I used to hate books. Now I choose not to live without them. Authors have become my spiritual counsellors, taking me to places and ideas that blow me away. Appointments are not necessary: my books are always there where I left them after my last visit; ready, willing and able to continue right where we left off. They're consistent: they're saying the same thing today as they did yesterday.

If I read an entire book and only one page resonates, that page has still enriched my life. The words on that one page will stay with me forever—all their meanings and influences lifting me on conscious and subconscious levels. I have developed this unquenchable thirst for knowledge and inspiration but I don't just roll over and accept every peabrained idea that I read. A pretty good system is in place to filter out the bullshit. The stuff that I connect with makes an immediate impact. The garbage is forgotten about immediately. I'm not going to waste my time trying to decipher nonsense. It's a new world I'm discovering but I'm wary of being a sucker for every half-baked attempt to explain the meaning of life. Ultimately, there's comfort in knowing other people have as many questions and obstacles in life as I do.

Take Nick Vujicic. Nick was born without arms or legs. He has only a small flipper of a foot to use for his phone, for writing emails, for keeping himself upright. He calls it his 'flipper foot'. When he was ten years old, Nick told his brother he wanted to end his life. He saw no prospects for happiness. He feared being a burden to his family for all his days. Nick decided that he would attempt to drown himself in his next nightly bath.

Now he's a globe-trotting visionary, using his story for good instead of self-pity, to get people to understand the joy that can be found in even the most difficult life. I look at Nick and my first thought is *Oh, the poor bastard.* But then you see what an optimistic, vibrant character he is and you realise a few of your own demons might be getting too much oxygen. There's nothing poor-bastard about Nick's character or self-esteem. If he's feeling like life is nothing but an incredible gift, what right do I have to worry? None.

The suicidal part of Nick's story is heartbreaking. I really do feel his pain. And then I really do feel the soaring high that has come from his recovery. Downsides are followed by even bigger upsides. *This too will pass.* It's the common thread in every inspirational story I've ever read or heard. Nick did get into the bath with the saddest of intentions. He couldn't go through with his plan, however, because he knew the grief it would cause his family. I love Nick's message of turning lemons into lemonade. Each of us are broken in some way. Nick has no limbs. Others among us have no morals, or have anger issues, negative lifestyles and attitudes that need to be recognised and modified. Which is worse?

Nick has this fantastic routine when he's speaking to children in schools. He's vertical, balancing on his flipper foot. He deliberately falls over on the table, right there in front of the kids. They gasp.

He has no arms to push himself up with. No feet, no legs. The children are looking at him, wondering what to do. Pick him up? Leave him there? Wait for the teacher to help? There's a bit of panic. Is he alright?

Nick is talking all the way through his performance. He says: 'Look, kids, don't freak out—this is what life is all about. Here's my example. I've fallen over but just you wait and see, I'll get back up. It might look impossible, but it's not.' He puts his forehead on the table, using his neck muscles to lift himself back upright. Look him up on YouTube. You'll see video clips that will bring you to tears. All our lives can be incredible if we're willing to break a few old habits. Nick isn't preaching without deep-seated knowledge. He's actually living the battle, every day of his life. Nick Vujicic is winning. Nick makes me want to live more optimistically and abundantly in spirit than I ever have before. He talks in every English-speaking country you can think of and the message always gets through because the message is universal. He's just so authentic.

> Our lives can be incredible if we're willing to break a few old habits.

When people meet him, they can't shake his hand because he doesn't have one to shake. He says to them with a big, broad smile: 'Come on, gimme a hug!' It's the same philosophy as David Mackenzie's: act warmly enough and it will rub off. There's no point shying away from Nick's differences. People are basically talking to a torso and a head. 'Come on, gimme a hug!'—I love that. It's wonderful. Nick might be missing a few odds and ends, but he has a heart. Perhaps it's the only possession that really matters.

Naked in Sydney

5 SEPTEMBER 2010, early morning: St Francis of Assisi is immune to the pain that would ordinarily be spearing through his system from bare, wounded feet. I'm oblivious to humiliation or embarrassment, above this mortal world. At no stage do I feel my behaviour is unreasonable or irrational. At no time do I react to the catcalling, tut-tutting and wolf-whistling coming my way. I ignore all attempts to intimidate or mock me. I am a higher being. Negativity is nonexistent. I am righteous and bold. I stride along George Street filled with the drive of divine purpose—but every time I approach someone, they run for the hills as if I'm a ghoul. I move away from George Street to trawl the back alleys, the homes of the homeless, the desperate and depraved. It's dark and deserted down here. A man could get himself killed. At no stage do I think it is strange that I have no clothes on.

I feel no fear amid the sadness and seediness, just extreme empathy for the down-and-out. They're everywhere, the skeletons of this world, the zombies, the living dead—and even they ignore me. Move along, they say, appalled by me. Beggars sleeping under newspapers and cardboard boxes scream at me: Get away! Get away! A decrepit old woman recoils. Who ever approaches her? No-one. Except to threaten or abuse her. Why aren't we all approaching her? Why doesn't every last one of us want to rescue her? The people who most need help, like that old woman, no-one goes near them. We can't even bear to look at her. Unperturbed, I go back to George Street, the mission still incomplete. I'm dismissed as a drunk even though I've never been so sober in my life.

Halfway up George Street, the bitter cold snaps me back to my senses. I am Craig Hamilton and I've been walking the main street of Sydney barefoot and naked for two hours. I have to get out of here. Nightmares are made of being exposed in public and I'm living it. Suddenly, my feet are red raw and sore. Every step is like treading on broken glass. I shouldn't be out here. I'm not really sure why I'm here . . . I walk another hundred metres . . . why am I here? . . . another hundred metres . . . I really shouldn't be here . . . another hundred metres . . . the pain is killing me. another hundred metres . . . I have to get back to my hotel now.

In the hotel foyer I ask myself: What in the hell are you doing? I cover myself the best I can, running to the lift, slamming the up button, bolting back along the corridor to my room—and . . . I don't have a key. Pockets have been in short supply. It's now five in the morning.

The pain from my sliced and diced feet is very real. I'm lucid enough to know I'm not well. Back in the lift, my fellow passengers are on their way to check out (and most likely never come back). You know those awkward moments in lifts when no-one speaks, everyone just staring at the numbers till you reach your floor? This is the awkward lift ride to top them all. In the foyer, I hurry over to reception and ask matter-of-factly: 'Can I have another key, please?'

'Of course, sir,' is the reply. 'Will there be anything else? Some clothes perhaps?' Standing there, I wonder why the staff just laugh as they hand over the key, rolling their eyes as if I'm a naughty schoolboy.

I have a very clear recollection of this night. Every last step. Mania isn't like being hypnotised and having the memory of your lunacy vanish at the click of fingers. The reaction of the staff baffles me to this day. Their lack of intervention and concern. Why didn't anyone try to stop me? Why didn't anyone ask if I needed help? And how can a man expose himself in public for two hours, in the heart of Sydney, without being arrested?

7 The Yogi and his message

Bad stuff can happen on the road to a better life, but it doesn't have to define us. If we use the pain to keep searching for answers we can find them, sometimes in truly amazing places. An enormous wooden bookcase sits next to my TV at home. It towers over our living room. The contents of the bookcase give me infinitely more pleasure than anything that comes out of the TV. *Autobiography of a Yogi*, by Paramahansa Yogananda, for instance, is phenomenal.

Paul Harragon, a former captain of the Newcastle Knights rugby league team, threw it in my lap at a time when my soul was crying. I was at the end of my tether and needed answers. I wanted to understand what I was going through and *why* I had to go through it at all. I had to know how it had come to this and, more to the point, how to wriggle free.

I had this unshakable sense that something vitally important was missing. *Autobiography of a Yogi* filled a hole, getting it into my thick head what a gift it is to simply be here. How much potential I might have, but how often I'm walking around as if I'm asleep. I see that in other people: what are we all waiting for? I look in the mirror: wake up!

Yogananda was a Hindu man whose words, thoughts and deeds

were so powerful that his legacy will live forever. His purpose was to get people to find their true selves without letting the ego take control of every situation. A whole new world opened up to me just from that very idea. The more I took Yogananda's advice and nourished my spirit, the better I felt. The better I felt, the more I wanted to nourish my spirit. What a beautiful not-so-vicious cycle to be caught up in.

For anyone flogging themselves twelve hours a day to put their kids through private school or get that new car, who knows that they're unhappy and struggling to cope, this book is for you, just as it was for me. The 600 pages of *Autobiography of a Yogi* were my first 600 steps to finding peace.

Yogananda talked about the opposite side of the coin from the one I was looking at. He told me to be content. Find my bliss. Make a conscious, determined decision to pursue the things I enjoy and shun the things that don't nurture the soul. He made me focus on the singular importance of being happy.

I had forgotten about it being the greatest objective of all. Be happy! It's the most important thing in the world, but how often do we consciously endeavour to make it happen? Trying to be happy should have dominated my thoughts, but for all the to-do lists and life plans I made, being happy wasn't on any of them. How ridiculous could I be? It should be at the top of every list, alongside 'Help our loved ones to find happiness'—they're so entwined.

> Be happy! It's the most important thing in the world, but how often do we consciously endeavour to make it happen?

My life until then had been all about gaining possessions and status. I appreciated Yogananda's message because he took Eastern beliefs and applied them to the Western world. He wasn't an

Indian yogi exclusively spending his time in New Delhi while telling the rest of the planet how to live. He went to the West. He went to the United States and taught yoga and meditation to the multitude of Americans battling their assortment of psychological issues. He showed them how Eastern philosophies could be of benefit while they still lived their regular lives of paying their bills, going to work, paying off the house, chasing their idea of the American Dream.

There's so much we can learn from the East. There's plenty the East can learn from us, too. It's about finding the middle ground. Quietening down the ego has been a huge step for me. It's nice to have the approval of others, but I'm realising that neediness is an obstacle to a good and fulfilling life.

8 Finding balance

I'm coming to understand 'happiness' isn't about trying to be wildly happy all the time, or never being sad—it's about balance.

How then do you achieve balance with bipolar? Understanding your own personal landscape is a huge help. My psychiatrist, Dr Alan Weiss, rates the fluctuating mood swings associated with bipolar disorder on a scale of minus-five to plus-five. Minus-five is clinically depressed, probably suicidal. Plus-five is manic, psychotic. Zero is where Dr Weiss wants me to be, smack-bang in the middle of the winding, twisting, turning road. But the problem, as anyone with bipolar will tell you, is that plus-one and plus-two are a whole lot of fun.

I must remind myself that plus-two can become plus-three in a heartbeat and with me, plus-three has shown a fondness for marching straight on through to the other side: plus-four and then full of momentum and recklessness, to where all hell breaks loose, plus-five. I've needed to understand that plus-three is already the beginning of mania. I've already let it go too far.

I look back at what happened at Broadmeadow, the whole heaven and hell scenario, how the emotions and feelings were so stark and real, and I never want to go there again. Coming down was a terrifying experience and one I don't wish to repeat any time soon. I love the saying about the difference between a religious person and a spiritual person: a religious person doesn't want to go to hell, while a spiritual person has already been there and doesn't want to go back. My memories of what felt like hell motivate me to search continually for balance, for zero, for the middle of the road.

Lows are more manageable than highs because when I'm down it's natural to seek elevation to a happier place. I pull back a bit on work, clear the decks of commitments, go for a massage, dive into one of the alternative therapies I've discovered (and will discuss later in this book). I'm less skilled at taking action against the elevated high, manic mood because it's a difficult addiction to kick.

The key has been understanding plus-two for what it is: a lie. Zero might sound numb and lifeless, but it isn't. I can still make zero very lively, thanks. I'm a fairly gregarious person anyway. The numbness that might be felt by others at ground zero is only relative to the addiction they've developed to the high. That has been the greatest lesson of all. Managing depression with bipolar disorder means controlling the high. If you reduce the chances of a trip high in the sky, it reduces the risk of the crippling depression that invariably follows.

It's like a reformed cocaine addict saying he feels numb now he's clean. He's not numb, he's just back to where he's supposed to be. Once I learned the power of zero, that *I* was in control when the scales of life were balanced, I started feeling free. Plus-two is not real happiness. It's a mirage, an illusion. All plus-two really wants to do is take me to plus-five and dump me there. I'm at my most sincerely happy when I'm on zero, trundling along in control, learning and discovering what I can. Faith and trust are crucial. I trust that everything will be alright if I just hang in there long enough. I don't need reminding of what can happen if I take my eye off the ball.

Anxieties, the obvious in-your-face dramas and the more subtle offshoots, can bring trouble as quickly as the sudden shock of a car crash. Managing my work–life balance is the key. Part of that has been reigning in the impact of (anti)social media. First rule of my fight-for-your-life club: no smartphone. I don't want a BlackBerry. I don't need an iPhone. They make it too easy to take work home. I'm protecting myself because I know how tempted I can be. With an iPhone or BlackBerry, there'd be no more putting my work bag down at the door and enjoying a night at home with the family.

I do not want an iLife. I want a real life.

I've got an old mobile phone, but it's perfect because you know what it can do? Make and receive phone calls. It's all I need. Home is for home, work is for work. We all need to learn to switch off.

9 Close your eyes and relax

Switching off in our 24/7 world is easier said than done, until you get into the way of it. Massage has become crucial to helping me switch off. More than 25 years ago I noticed a sign on the noticeboard at my gym that said remedial massage could help with sports injuries. Cut to two and a half decades later and nearly 30 years of playing cricket had left me with back, elbow, knee and shoulder complaints. I can still remember the first appointment I made for remedial massage. I was asked which parts of my body needed attention. My back, I told the therapist. She asked if I would like a relaxation massage as well. I was pretty stressed at this stage. I said, 'Give me every kind of massage you've got.'

'Terrific. Now undress down to your underwear.'

I was thinking, OK, what's going on here? I have to be half naked? I am actually quite comfortable being naked, it's really not such a big deal . . . but you have to pick your place. (The streets of Sydney in the middle of winter is not the place.) But I stripped down to my undies and soon learned there was nothing to worry about. They put towels around me and only worked on the parts of my body that needed attention. Mainly my back, shoulders and neck, which really hold a lot of tension.

The relaxation effect is supreme. The relief may be only temporary, but it's relief nonetheless and I'll take whatever relief I can get, for as long as it lasts when I'm hurting. Cost can be a factor, but I'm happy to splurge on massage when I'm feeling really anxious or agitated. I leave every session thinking it's been worth every cent. The touch of a trained human hand can be incredibly comforting when you're distressed.

An hour-long session feels like six hours when I'm sliding into such deep relaxation. I completely switch off, escape the negative thoughts that have dragged me through the door in the first place. Weekly sessions give me something to look forward to. I like the regularity of the appointments. It's a reason to get out of the house when I'm tempted to stay inside and mope.

The length of the post-massage boost depends on how severe the symptoms have been to start with. With moderate depression, I'll get two weeks of tangible benefit. In the grip of the most severe depression, I might only get relief for the rest of that day. Next morning, I'm back on the low road—but still convinced it's been worth the expense. I've been able to see through the fog for another day, which means I'm another day closer to coming out the other side.

10 What next?

To help keep myself on an even keel, I've learned to watch out for those times when I'm going over the limit. You can feel when you're going over the limit. Initial feelings of curiosity become desperate searches for more. We've all been there. The dishes are piled up in the kitchen, the kids need to be put to bed, you know you should log off but just can't. The little red light on the laptop keeps flashing with the temptation of something new. I know people who spend all day and night on computers and telephones. If it's for work, I get it. But it's never all for work. No-one needs to work that much. You finish your shift but decide it's better to do some more work at home.

What a waste of an hour. Get a life. That's what I ended up telling myself. I needed to drop the nonsense that I was doing the right thing by taking my work home. You're doing right by your boss, maybe, but wrong by everyone else, including your parents, partner or children. They want to talk to you. They don't want to watch you use an app. Who's more important? Your family or your boss?

My bosses want me ready for work in the morning in the best state I can be. They want me on song for that shift, no more and no less. They want me fresh and alert. If I'm doing all this other rubbish the night before, I'll be no good the next day. What takes me two hours to get through at night will take just 30 minutes when I'm fresh the next morning. Burnout is my concern. The favourite button on my phone is the one which switches the bloody thing off. We're supposed to be the laidback nation but that's becoming a myth. Most of us are working 50, 60-plus hours a week. My question is this: for what? Oh, if I could get back the lost time.

I was a dedicated sports commentator, but less devoted to my duties as father and husband. I judged myself by my material successes and failures, and by my professional status. It took a while to realise they were *perceived* successes and failures. My performances as husband and father should've been the real gauge of my worth. False gods had taken over. Work is impor-tant, but it was too important. Check out all the tombstones in the cemetery. None of them say: 'HERE LIES JOE BLOGGS, HE WISHES HE'D SPENT MORE TIME AT THE OFFICE.'

I know a bloke who demolished a perfectly good house and replaced it with a sprawling two-storey home. The new place has a pool in the backyard, two bathrooms, five bedrooms—all brand new. From the outside, it looks great, fit for a king. His life appears to be going ahead in leaps and bounds, but I don't see him any more. The success is an illusion. There's no socialising and no real friendships because he's working morning, noon and night to pay the bills. I imagine he's miserable as well as invisible.

The opposite scenario is the guy three doors down from him. He's had the same block of land for close to 30 years—and the same old house. He's done some renovating over the years but never felt the need to extend or knock it down. It's his house and he's happy in it. He works normal hours for a normal salary and he's content. I know which of those two blokes is better off.

Problem is, we all have a desire to be loved, admired and respected—but we don't know how to achieve it. I used to think

I had to work harder and constantly achieve for affection to be thrown my way. I fell into thinking I'd be appreciated and more if I acquired additional material wealth and career upgrades. Einstein said: 'Try not to become a man of success but rather to become a man of value.' Hear, hear.

Once I cultivated the image of outrageous fortune. Now I know I could be growing chokos for a living and my family and real friends would like me just as much as if I was curing cancer (or bipolar). More importantly, I would still like myself just as much. Those who don't, well, I'm better off without them anyway. Real friendships are all I'm interested in. Love and support should be unconditional. The sad part of the guy working twelve hours a day is that he's *trying* to do the right thing. Everyone tells him how proud they are of him. Oh, what a trouper. He's trying to improve himself and his life, but I think his energies are misguided.

Workaholics need to be pointed in the right direction. In 2011 a survey by Just Better Care, an organisation that enables ill or elderly people to remain living at home, found more Australians over the age of 65 were worried about money (23 per cent) than their health (20 per cent) and families (19 per cent). Spare me, please! Something is seriously amiss when people in the glorious twilight of their life are fretting about how much cash they have in the bank.

I thank my good friend Barry Smith for giving me a small book by Spencer Johnson called *The Precious Present*. The title says it all—what a great gift. Barry saw very clearly what I could not. I used to be obsessed with 'What's next?' It meant I could never sit still. No time to waste, got to keep moving: onwards and upwards, onwards, more upwards. I needed to be *still*, catch my breath, look around and make proper plans instead of shooting off in all directions.

The constant striving tore me away from where
I should have been: in the present moment.

I did start making more money and acquired extra possessions. Really, they changed nothing. I could've had the biggest mansion in Australia overlooking the entire Newcastle skyline but nothing would have improved in my most important section of real estate: the fifteen centimetres between my ears.

I really don't want to sound as if I'm preaching from an ivory tower because I still have struggles. I've made some changes to my life that have been victories but I still get dragged back to the bad old days because I do live in the Western world. I do hold down a job. I do need to provide for my family, and I still have a mortgage. All things I can't just walk away from.

We all have commitments of one sort or another. We can't just pretend they don't exist and say see you later, I'm off to sit under a tree in the Himalayas and meditate for the rest of my life. Well, I suppose I could, but I choose not to. I want the best of both worlds. Please don't think I'm endorsing quitting work. I just think more of us need to manage our lives in a reasonable and sensible way. Providing for a family goes beyond financial contributions.

When working was my top priority, when I thought about it endlessly, I was forever tired. Endlessly cranky. Relationships in my own family started suffering. I could feel it happening but in a strange way, I couldn't stop it. I used work as an excuse, kidding myself I was doing great by everyone.

Quality time became non-existent. Free time was devoted to recovering from all the work I'd just done, or getting ready for the next shift. It could never last. I hardly saw friends outside work. I was rarely home to see Louise and the kids. There could be no perfect result because the pursuit itself was so imperfect.

The obsession to achieve, to earn a bigger wage, to keep up with all the Joneses (there's a few of them), the endless pursuit of 'What's next?' was too much. I'd created this persona of someone who was successful in the media. My ego was being fed and the bigger it got, the more expectation I put on myself to keep it growing and expanding. I fell into the trap of wanting more, more, more; running around at top speed trying to achieve everything at once, exhausting myself and all those diving for cover around me. Curbing 'What's next?' has been, and remains to this day, the greatest challenge. People who run around at a million miles an hour, I call them flappers. I was flapping so hard I fell in a screaming heap on a train platform. All I was really doing was staying where I was, arms going fast, me going nowhere. I'm a reformed flapper.

11 Hands off!
The power of reiki

When you set off on your quest to find a better way of living, it's amazing how many different ways you can support your health and who you really want to be. Reiki, literally a hands-off form of healing, has been an important part of this. That wasn't my initial response to the experience, I have to admit.

My first thought was: Why am I wasting money on this? The therapist isn't even touching my skin! See, witchcraft. It seemed absurd. I'm lying on a bed, face up—and the therapist is working five centimetres above my body! Waving her hands around, up and down, from head to toe. I'm lying there thinking: You know, I work pretty hard for my dough. And I'm throwing it away on this?

I really did think it was ridiculous but, because I had already paid, I decided I was going to make the practitioner work for every last cent, so I stuck at it. Straight after the session, I felt fantastic. It was a sensation that lasted for days afterwards. The edge had disappeared entirely. The first little miracle.

You're fully clothed as opposed to stripping off for a massage. That might be of comfort to some people. Reiki can either be hands-on from the practitioner or, amazingly, as I've said, hands-off. Reiki concentrates on different meridian points of the body.

A hand might be placed on or above the solar plexus, heart, leg, knee, on the chest. It might be on the third eye chakra right in the middle of your forehead, or on the top of your head. The therapy is energy based, directing it around the body, blasting away blockages caused by trauma, freeing up areas of tension.

Psychological issues can manifest themselves in physical problems. Memories of trauma or just plain old stress can cause it. The feeling is real, you know it, but the only way you can deal with the issues is to put them in a box, close the lid and never open it again. I think the gremlins inside us don't like to be ignored. It's as if they have to be acknowledged before they'll agree to disappear. Reiki works on the parts of the body where these traumas have revealed themselves in a physical way. Having a therapist work five centimetres above the body sounds mad, I know, but it really has left me with renewed clarity and calm.

12 Discovering Philip Yancey

Philip Yancey has been another revelation. He's a Christian writer with a difference—because he's a Christian writer with doubts. More to the point, he's a Christian who *admits* to having doubts. I appreciate his honesty. I'm not interested in blind faith on any topic. No-one enjoys being hit over the head with ideas. I'm interested in someone pointing out the possibilities then leaving me to my own devices. I wouldn't call myself a believer but I hesitate to call myself a non-believer because quotes like this from C. S. Lewis—'God is sculpting us every day and shaping us into what we are destined to become'—most definitely strike a chord. I'm just not sure what the chord is. I want to make up my own mind and Yancey makes me feel free to do that. He's sold an incredible number of books, more than 14 million. His titles reveal the extent of the internal warfare going on: *What Good is God?*, *What's So Amazing About Grace?*, *The Jesus I Never Knew*, *Disappointment with God*, *Church: Why Bother?*

He has painful moments when the doubts overwhelm him. But then he has doubts about the doubts, too, with stages of great conviction. He's saying there is *something* out there, so let's go investigate. I think that's brilliant. Philip Yancey believes the spiritual side of life is genuine, but he's also brave enough to admit he doesn't fully grasp the intricacies. I like the fact that Yancey has the same questions as I do. He says the power of the church is weakened by trying to force everyone to adopt its views. I respect him enormously for that, too. Yancey makes me feel as if we're on the same path.

I might be 3000 miles behind him in experience and insight; I might be 5000 miles further back, but he makes me feel like we're on the same road to recovery nonetheless. He's welcoming anyone to join the conversation at any time and with whatever views we may have. I appreciate his honesty. He makes me think I don't need to wait for a life emergency to start asking the big questions. If I decide spirituality is garbage and I want to take the off ramp, Yancey tells me I should do it. The feeling is that *something* is out there, guiding us along. I don't know what that something is but the more I embrace the possibility—even probability—of its existence, the more alive I feel. The more *right* I feel, as if the real me is coming out. I love the thought of an alternate reality, one lifting us free from negativity and doubt and fear, guiding us away from troubles if we only believe in it. It might be a belief in God, the perfection that exists in the universe, or karma. The thought that our existence is some random fluke does not wash with me. Call it evolution if you like but, whatever it is, we are all in the game.

Yancey's big questions fascinate me. What are we doing here? What's the point of these lives of ours? Anything on the other side? Heaven? Hell? God? Any kind of spirit world? Ghosts? Dreams? Was Jesus physically resurrected or was he just a human being (without doubt one of the most influential men who ever lived) who died on a cross? Was his body dragged out by his friends and, three days later, someone thought they saw him (or someone who looked like him) and that's how the story began? My answer to all these questions used to be 'Who cares?'.

Now my answer is 'Tell me more'. The more I read and learn, the more I want to read and learn. I've become a *voracious* reader. This *something* I feel, what is it?

13 Dark nights of the soul

In spite of all the good work you put in, it doesn't mean you'll never suffer again. What it does mean is that you've got a ready-made set of tools for picking yourself up. You can only do this when you're prepared to realise you're not in great shape.

It's hard to talk about the down times, because they can take you a long way down. Depression isn't something any of us like to focus on. In fact, stories about depression stop me cold. What I've found, however, is that it can be really helpful to learn from those who have been there before you. Gifted writers are putting into words what I have experienced myself. They could not be more accurate if I'd told them myself. Hundreds of people, thousands of people, millions of people are trying to get a grip on the same issues. That's a little overwhelming, to think about the global scale, but incredibly settling to know someone has been through it and lived to tell the tale. I feel like I'm a member of this huge, sprawling club, the author and myself and the hordes of people reading the same pages as me. I can picture us all flicking through the same books at the same time.

Thomas Moore's *Dark Nights of the Soul* is incredibly confronting. His descriptions of clinical depression mirror precisely my own recollections. But he writes: 'A dark night of the soul can heal, where healing means being more alive and more present to the world around you.' It's a tough book to read because it reminds me of the whole manifestation of depression and how much of a beating it gives me. It's as if the life force inside me has been stolen and hidden where I can't find it. Colours don't look colourful; warmth doesn't feel warm; cold doesn't feel cold; uplifting songs sound sad . . . there's just nothing worthwhile in anything. The more harrowing the read, however, the more powerful the message of perseverance.

Dark Nights of the Soul moved me so much that I wrote Thomas Moore a letter and sent him a copy of my first book, *Broken Open*. About six months later, to my utter astonishment, an envelope arrived in my mailbox with a US postmark on it. Thomas Moore had replied. 'What a wonderful book,' he wrote. 'You have turned a challenging situation into a lifelong passion where you can help others.' I'm not too shy to admit that was pretty terrific. I felt validated in what I was trying to do, and still do. His letter has found a home in the manila folder. It reminds me I am on the right track when I do need reminding.

I don't show too many people the letter from Thomas Moore because I imagine them rolling their eyes and thinking, 'Put it away and stop being such a bloody show-off!' One of the few people I have shown it to is my first cousin, Faith. She's aptly named because Faith, now gracefully moving through her 60s, has been a Sister of Mercy since the age of eighteen. One day when Faith visited our home I pulled Thomas Moore's letter out of the drawer and showed her. She didn't say much, to be honest. She was probably rolling her eyes and thinking I should stop being such a bloody show-off.

14 Show some respect

Throughout this whole process I've come to realise that every part of every person's journey matters—the good bits and the hard bits. That's something we can easily forget in the celebrity-driven culture we're in. I'm continually amazed at the courage shown by people from all walks of life who are dealing with their demons as well as their dreams. It's important we show respect regardless of how hard the journey gets, as this moving letter reminds us.

> My mother suffered from depression. We would often come home to find her crying uncontrollably for no apparent reason and we watched her suffer more than one nervous breakdown during her lifetime. I have also lost a 21-year-old relative to suicide for this very reason, so well done—for your bravery, for your fighting spirit and your gutsy, honest way. I've always regarded you highly, but you are an absolute hero in my eyes now.

When you read this letter the heroism shines through. Let's be honest, I reckon American country music legend Johnny Cash and David Mackenzie were heroes. One was famous; the other was not. With their vastly different tales, they prove heroes can emerge from anywhere at any time. For small or large reasons.

Once Johnny Cash was recording an album at a studio. He was already a huge star. When no-one was watching, he could have been looking out only for himself. The janitor at the studio where Johnny Cash recorded some of his biggest hit records liked to sit in on his sessions.

One day a couple of musicians crashed the session. The secretary to the producer blamed the janitor, telling him he wasn't allowed into the session that night. Instead he had to stay in the basement and do his work. He did as he was told, quietly going about his business. Johnny Cash went down to see him: 'I heard you're not coming up to my recording session tonight.'

The janitor said, 'Yeah, there's work I need to do down here.'

Johnny Cash said, 'Well, I'm just telling you, unless you're up there watching me tonight, I won't be recording anything.'

So the janitor went up and watched. The secretary was so cranky she was glaring at the janitor the whole session. That janitor was Kris Kristofferson before *he* was a star. You might say, so what? Big deal. But Kristofferson never forgot. He still tells that story during his shows to illustrate the impact of all our deeds.

People are fascinating. All of them. I love the thought that I'm just one piece of the universal puzzle. It's fascinating to track human history and it stops me getting bogged down in my own little world. There are six billion of us roaming round and what an amazing experience this all is. I like that Johnny Cash story: his heart was for the battler.

15 Hang on to your dreams

I've discovered that part of lasting the journey is holding onto your dreams. Of the five major dreams I've had in my life, the most rewarding is the one I'm living right now.

The first dream was to play tennis at Wimbledon. Dad suggested the novel idea of trying my luck at the local courts at Howe Park first. I did everything I could to become the best tennis player I could be. Wimbledon was just pie in the sky: I was so young, I wouldn't have minded being Superman, either. The All England Club was going to be a couple of Sundays too far away for this little baseline slugger. The older we get, the more realistic the dreams become. My next fantasy lasted a good twelve years. I was going to play Test cricket for Australia.

I started receiving recognition as a cricketer when I was fifteen. I was picked in the Singleton Under Sixteens and thought I was on my way. I moved to Newcastle, one of the strongest sporting nurseries in Australia, and made the Newcastle XI. Test players have come from that team: Gary Gilmour, Rick McCosker and Robert 'Dutchy' Holland. When I was chosen for NSW Country, the goal was still very real—but fading fast. I played against Sri Lanka at McKitrick Park at Grafton. Half-a-dozen Test stars were in the Sri Lankan team and I held my own.

From my grainy memory, my bowling figures that day were nine overs, three maidens, 0–28, but you can never be too sure about these things! This dream wasn't so unrealistic. It was still in my mind and still a goal: I *can* do this. Realistically I was miles away but in your dreams you can always aim high. But then came the decline. I was dropped from NSW Country team, I was dropped from the Newcastle XI. Another dream was over. No worries, I'd done my best. When one dream ends, you just go grab another.

The third dream was to become a sports commentator. Bingo! But it was a million miles away. I was working in a coalmine. My experience of sports commentary amounted to blow-by-blow accounts of backyard games with my brother Ian, when we were younger, and imaginary calls of NRL games while I was down the mine. In other words, I had no experience at all. The thought of working for the ABC was patently ridiculous, but so what? I could still have the goal. The great thing about dreams is that there are no limits.

When one dream ends, you just go grab another.

I kept my dream to myself. With anything you really want to achieve, something you hold especially dear to your heart, keep it sacred until it happens. Hang on to it. They're private thoughts, they're all yours and, anyway, it's fun to be on your own private mission. Never let go of the dream until there's absolutely definitive proof you've picked something unattainable. Be careful when you pull the pin. It doesn't matter what someone else thinks about your goals and aspirations, it's what you think that counts.

If you start telling everyone what you want to do, the nay-sayers will come from everywhere: 'Wake up to yourself! You'll never do that. It's just not possible. It'll never happen.

You're kidding yourself!' Don't let them drag you down. My dream of commentary was only fulfilled through sheer persistence and ignoring those who told me to quit. It took seven years to sign a contract for full-time employment with ABC Radio. If I can go from being down a coalmine to sitting next to Steve Mortimer, Warren Ryan, Peter Wilkins or David Morrow in an ABC Radio commentary box, practically anything can happen.

I thank Peter Wilkins for his fantastic mentoring at this stage of my career. Wilko is one of the true professionals and gave me the confidence to really have a crack at this broadcasting caper, and I learned plenty from him.

The Olympics was the next dream. We all know how that ended: quickly, emphatically and bluntly. I figured I might as well do something with the diagnosis, to find out if some good could come from what initially seemed all bad. So the fifth and biggest and most satisfying dream of all, to help others see the hidden gifts, has kicked in *because* of bipolar. It is such hard work, which makes all the more worthwhile. I don't want a soft and comfortable life. I want these challenges.

> If I can go from being down a coalmine to sitting next to Steve Mortimer, Warren Ryan, Peter Wilkins or David Morrow in an ABC Radio commentary box, practically anything can happen.

Perhaps I should thank bipolar for giving me the opportunity to stop being such a selfish bastard. If I could nominate one word to encapsulate my view on the meaning of life, the one action guaranteed to make me feel like the stars have aligned, it would be this: *helping*. Spreading the word about mental health has made me feel more spiritually rewarded than any other pursuit. It's as if the bipolar and all the back-breaking struggles are actually helping me serve my purpose in life. No more flapping. Curiously enough, since I've consciously started putting life ahead of work, the biggest beneficiary has been work.

16 Medication—a vital part of the jigsaw

Personal experience has taught me that I *must* take medication.

Alternative therapies are invaluable and life-enhancing, but the nuts and bolts of treating bipolar disorder is the medication. I realise how important it is and am thankful for what it does. Please don't think that all you have to do to treat bipolar is get off the drink, do a few yoga classes, take a 9.5 kilometre walk and Bob's your father's brother. The fact is, without medication, I'm in trouble. Paul Dudley White, the late American physician and cardiologist, said: 'A vigorous five-mile walk will do more good for an unhappy but otherwise healthy adult than all the medicine and psychology in the world.' That's true, but when the mental wellbeing of the person involved falls under the category of 'it's complicated', there is an imbalance, and daily medication is the most important piece in the jigsaw puzzle of managing bipolar. The other regimes are the back-up troops.

I take 1000 milligrams of the mood-stabilising drug Epilim (sodium valproate) every night. I also take 100 milligrams daily of Lamictal (lamotrigine), an anticonvulsive medication which is also an effective mood stabiliser. I take 50 milligrams in the morning and 50 milligrams at night. My psychiatrist, Dr Weiss, has had terrific results with bipolar patients on this medication.

It should be put on the Pharmaceutical Benefits Scheme (PBS). At the time of writing, patients are paying top dollar for it, meaning too many cannot afford it. (Ludicrously, you can claim Lamictal on the PBS if it is prescribed to treat convulsions but not to control bipolar.)

Another medication which should be on the PBS is Valdoxan (agomelatine). Dr Weiss put me on this melatonin-based anti-depressant as soon as it came out, and it has been very effective in helping to regulate my sleep patterns, a vital part of managing bipolar. I have 25 milligrams every night. It helps to get the circadian rhythm back to a normal range, because that's one thing that goes out the window in depression. When I was in a bad way in September 2010 I had a hard time sleeping, but after two or three days of taking Valdoxan, I was sleeping like a log. It didn't remove the depression but the restored sleep pattern was a blessing.

Mental health treatment shouldn't depend on prosperity. I'm in the fortunate enough position of being able to afford the drugs I need, but I know plenty of people who aren't. It costs me $140 a month to stay on both Valdoxan and Lamictal. How is anyone who is unemployed or on a basic wage with three kids and a mortgage going to afford that? The answer is they can't. That creates a vicious cycle which starts with a mental illness, which may lead to hospitalisation where the illness is stabilised, then to discharge and an inability to pay for the medications used in hospital . . . so it's back to square one.

People are missing out on treatments that could be hugely beneficial to their health simply because they're living too close to the breadline. That's a tragedy. I know exactly what can happen next, because it's happened to me: Not taking my medication leaves me vulnerable to severe episodes of mania.

I cannot emphasise it enough: I must be vigilant with my medication. It is so critical to taking the edge off the highs and the lows. It gives more time to act and intervene before the situation gets out of hand. If you have two or three days before you drop into the pit, instead of two or three hours, there's more chance of avoiding the pit altogether.

Medication is no guarantee against depression or mania but it's as close as we can get. Alternative therapies can play an important role, but medication is the first and most important piece of the puzzle. Without it, all the alternative therapies in the world aren't going to make much difference. They're the top-up, the icing on the cake.

For my first seven years with bipolar, from the very first day I was sent home after the railway experience in 2000, I took one medication only. I was taking 1500 milligrams per day of Epilim, and that did the job for those seven years. Since then, however, with more episodes, my medication has required tweaking.

With any psychological illness, there are very few people who don't go through periods of adjusting their medication. When I've been high in more recent times, I've been medicated with Zyprexa (olanzapine), another very useful mood stabiliser, very effective in reining in the high. Dr Weiss throws me on that for a short period, until the symptoms disappear again. At times when I have a small high which runs the risk of escalating, I'll have 2.5 milligrams of Zyprexa added to my medication.

When I was hospitalised in 2010, when I was manic, I was put on 30 milligrams a day. That's a big whack with some pretty significant sedative powers. It's been terrifically effective for me. They're the only medications I've been on. (I'm currently off Zyprexa, but it can be added when required.)

I'm very tuned into the fact that medication is impor-tant. Any lapses are accidental, and only ever for one night. For example, I might crash out in front of the TV before I've meant to, woken up and it's the next morning. But I'm straight back on the program the next day and there's no damage done. Isolated slip-ups aren't the problem. The danger is in the kind of complacency that will make you skip medication for weeks on end. I had a stage where I refused to stick with Lamictal because I told Dr Weiss it simply wasn't working. He wanted me to have another try and in the past twelve months I have been taking it, the difference in my health has been noticeable.

You might be on holidays and feel fantastic. I've been like that. Why do I need to be medicated? I feel great! But every missed day is another small chip in the wall. One minor crack won't matter. It can be covered up, pronto. But stay lazy and I'll be in trouble. There can be no complacency, none. I *must* medicate.

A painful dose of reality

5 SEPTEMBER 2010: Back in my hotel room, I slam the door shut. It's nearly 5 a.m. Seven hours have passed since I first crawled in here. The sun will be up soon, sticking its head in to see what the hell has been going on. I call home and tell Louise we're on again. Send the cavalry. It really is happening again.

I'm delusional when Louise arrives with her friend, Kim. From just before 5 a.m., when I had just enough clarity to know I needed to make the call, to when they arrived at 7 a.m., I pace around outside my hotel room, still half-naked, my mind spinning with all sorts of wild ideas— manic and delusional, if marginally less psychotic.

Louise and Kim turn up about 7.30 a.m. Kim needs to be here, she's right to be here, she's a great family friend—but I shoot her a look and snap, 'You shouldn't be here, Kim. This is none of your damn business, this is private.' Louise sits me down. She sees the mad look in my eyes. She tries to bring me back to reality: 'Craig, I want to talk to you. What are you thinking?'

I tell her that she knows very well what I'm thinking: 'Don't give me that rubbish. You don't even need to ask. You know who I am.'

She's saying, 'Who are you? Who are you, Craig?'

I keep saying, 'You know who I am, you know who I am!'

She gives me four Risperidone, a powerful antipsychotic medication.

This dose is enough to knock out a herd of elephants. We're in the car going to the nearest hospital and the drugs aren't working yet. I'm still as high as a kite, talking nonstop, laughing too loud at what aren't even jokes: 'This is great! This is the best ride I've ever been on! I feel like we're on a roller-coaster! Yahoo!'

We get to Emergency and the drugs start kicking in. I'm drowsy and then I'm out like a light. Louise tells the nurse she would rather take me home to Newcastle than stay in Sydney. She assures the nurse she can get me back to Newcastle, to family and familiarity and home sweet home, in one piece. Then she rings the ABC and tells them I won't be into work for a while.

I sleep most of the way back to Newcastle, waking now and again to make some inane comment, so inane that Louise tells me to shut up and go back to sleep. Louise is acting tough, and she is tough, but who knows what she's really thinking. Am I OK? Time will tell. When I'm assessed at James Fletcher Hospital, there's no sign of mania or an elevated mood or psychosis because she's banged me up with so much Risperidone.

17 When blokedom doesn't help

I've mentioned my reluctance to tell Steve Mortimer I wasn't OK at Parramatta Stadium. The reason for that was 'blokedom'. It's a conditioned and dangerous state. As Australian males, we're taught by our families to be resilient and tough. To avoid showing our emotions under any circumstances. We have been conditioned to think it's a sign of weakness if we do. We must battle on regardless, be stoic and fight the good fight—without any help. These traits can help us to a point, but our women are supposed to be the ones bringing the emotion to the table.

We're supposed to be the rocks, the troupers, the unbreakable soldiers. This expectation has existed since day one because the nation itself was forged in harsh terrain and on a certain survival of the fittest. Even today, kudos is given to men who keep going even when they're unwell. We're supposed to be ironmen, tough as teak, rugged and invincible. Men's men. If worst comes to worst, we should *pretend* we're OK because that's preferable to showing sensitivity or vulnerability.

If most blokes are being deeply honest with themselves, they'll admit to the pressure of having to prove themselves a man, especially when it comes to their physique, their jobs and their health. This pressure doesn't happen by itself. Our boys are taught to be strong and independent from a young age—before they've learned who they are as a person and what works for them. It's so sad, because it creates men who will go to extraordinary lengths to prove they don't need help, when with a little intervention their lives could be a thousand times better. Put a bloke in a macho environment and the pressure on him goes up 1000 per cent. For some this environment is toxic, for others it can be lethal. This was really brought home to me in a moving letter:

> Living in a mining town for 30 years, and being a long-term union delegate, I've seen the results too many times of our failure to realise that mental illness is just that. An illness like any other. It's not weak or self-indulgent to get one. Hard work, too much grog, workplace bullying, isolation, constant pressure, family strife, marriage breakdown, pressure to be harder and stronger than perhaps we know in our own minds that we are, all can contribute to pushing people past their limit. In the workplace we are only just now starting to deal with these issues.
>
> In the old days, not too long ago, the person simply disappeared from site, never to be seen again. Now, with the help and understanding of their workmates and a reluctant management, people are getting well and returning to work, albeit after a lengthy break. This is because people like yourself are talking about it and explaining it to others. Also, we can see that it is treatable and that there is life after it. What you are doing makes the job of support persons so much easier.

What I see is that the more macho the industry, the more likelihood of trouble. All that pressure to be Superman. I think about this: what would have happened if I'd been diagnosed while working down the mines instead of working for the ABC? I think it would have been a whole different story. Possibly a much more tragic tale: I might not have survived. That isn't a criticism of the coal industry as it is today, because the culture in that rough-and-tumble industry, and many others, is greatly

improved. The modern coal industry is really making a difference for its employees by educating them about mental health.
But that wasn't the case when I was down the pit. I left the coal
industry in 1997. If the events of 2000 had happened ten years
earlier, I don't know where I'd be now. I don't know if I'd be
here at all.

The level of misunderstanding at the time may well have
denied me the support I needed. I would not have recovered
as well, if at all. I probably would have lost my job and never
been heard from again. That was the fate of many a poor soul in
the dark old days. One day a bloke was working, next day they
were reported ill, sent to hospital, gone from the site and no-one
knew why. That wasn't just in the coal industry, it was part of
society. The victims were glad to vanish, no questions asked, to
save themselves the embarrassment of admitting what they had
fallen victim to.

Being different was viewed less favourably back then. It's
fantastic that these days miners aren't hung out to dry. One of
the great advancements I've seen in the last decade is that the coal
industry is becoming proactive instead of reactive about mental
health issues. I've done presentations for a number of the big coal
companies. They want their employees to receive mental health
information: if they're briefed, if the issue is on the table with
employers and employees getting an overview of the issue before
something does come up, that's a major step forward in awareness. If progress can be made in as tough an industry as this, it
could and should be happening everywhere. Cultures can change
quickly if there's enough determination.

18 Changing the status quo

If we want things to change for men we need to make some changes ourselves. Rightly or wrongly or ruinously it's the way we're programmed, or the way we program ourselves: the strong, silent, macho types are admired. They conquer life and women and any obstacle. We crush beer cans with our bare hands, eat raw meat. When depressions and fragilities arise, which they do in every single one of us, even if to varying degrees, we become ashamed and retreat to our caves. It's an extension of the significance we attach to those all-important outward appearances.

> 'Pay no attention to what critics say. No statue has ever been erected to a critic.'
>
> Jean Sibelius

My happiness used to depend entirely on what everyone else thought of me. What a waste of my time and energy. Now I realise what anyone else thinks about me is none of my business. I can see, late in my life but not too late, that self-respect is more valuable than the respect of a hundred others. I spend more time with me than anyone else. I spend *all* my time with me. I need us to get along. It's the most important relationship I have with direct consequences for every other one I have.

Fighting the good fight alone is fine, but some problems are just too big to handle on your own. Different people have different ways of coping with mental illness but I really doubt it can be done alone. Blokedom is a common thread among the tragic, life-ending stories of mental illness, of which there are many. Not every patient admitted to psychiatric hospitals gets out alive. We would rather die than admit to our shortcomings. The raw and dangerous emotions of mental illness can become buried under too much alcohol, drug taking, excessive gambling, too much commitment to work—any number of addictions. Anything to avoid admitting or finding the truth.

They are all a con: man-made solutions to nature-based problems, unable to permanently protect us from what is really gnawing away. Think of a termite eating away at your house. Deal with it early and the house is saved. Ignore it and hope it goes away, hope it will miraculously disappear if you don't mention it and pretend it doesn't exist, and the walls will come crashing down.

Addictions are just coping mechanisms to mask the uncomfortable nature of certain realities. As Australian men, we have to be brave enough to acknowledge our most acute problems. If we don't, eventually, they will make their presence felt and the longer we've been in denial, the more severe the final explosion will be. Trust me on that, and this: manhood has nothing to do with staying quiet. It has everything to do with having the balls to speak up.

> It took every ounce of my strength to give the impression I was coping when really, I wasn't coping at all.

I find it difficult to get rid of my blokedom. I was taught never to cry, never to ask for help, to put on a brave face and never to show emotional weaknesses. This is just the way it was for men of my generation and the generations before that. It took every ounce of my strength to give the impression I was coping when really, I wasn't coping at all. Impressions: who cares? I want realities. I thought I couldn't tell anyone about my depression, not even Louise, even when I knew she would want to know because then she could help. I was too ashamed and embarrassed about the way I was feeling. I thought everyone would think less of me, and abandon me, so I locked everyone out and curled up in my cave. Suffering was preferable to having people's opinions change. That was idiotic. No-one had any idea how bad the situation was until I was crippled with clinical depression and had suicidal thoughts midway through 2000.

In a way, once the mushroom cloud of dust had settled, it was a relief. 'Remember that not getting what you want is sometimes a wonderful stroke of luck,' says the Dalai Lama. Luck came in the form of no longer having to pretend. Play-acting had been exhausting in itself. Blokedom is unhealthy enough to have a definite link to depression and, in my case, bipolar.

> 'Not getting what you want is sometimes a wonderful stroke of luck.'
>
> His Holiness the Dalai Lama

It's changing, though, slowly but surely, because prominent, trailblazing Australian men such as Andrew Johns and Wally Lewis have revealed their experiences. These are extremely successful guys. You could have a beer with them at your local pub and think they had life sorted out better than anyone. Again, outward appearances are never worth much. By telling their stories, these guys are empowering others, including me, to get a handle on our own situations. Says AFL legend Wayne Schwass: 'I manage to stay healthy with a combination of exercise, eating a balanced diet and having little or no alcohol—but the greatest thing I have done for myself is telling those closest to me about my condition. Being open and honest has been the single most important thing I have done for my own health and wellbeing.'

Andrew and Wally, two of the all-time greats of rugby league, have been at the forefront of the march out of the caves. They're among the toughest athletes Australia has ever produced, dominating one of the most brutal sporting contests in the country, State of Origin. Both have battled mental illness. Both have shared their stories. It's difficult to measure how many people they have helped by being so honest about their experiences. They've shattered the notion that staying silent is remotely connected to toughness because these two, without any shred of doubt, are as tough as they come. In the past, when mental health issues appeared, Australian men tried to work it out for ourselves because that's what we've thought we were supposed to do. It's what our heroes did. Now the heroes are taking a different route.

Anzac Day

ANZAC DAY. One of my hardest lessons came on 25 April 2007. I'm driving my son, Josh, from Newcastle to the Sydney Football Stadium for the clash between the Sydney Roosters and St George Illawarra Dragons. I will be watching and talking from the ABC commentary booth. Josh will be watching the game from the grandstand. We never arrive.

I'm driving steadily towards the link road to the F3 that will take us from Newcastle to Sydney, in torrential rain. It happens very quickly for something I can still replay in slow motion if I close my eyes. One minute, everything is great, we're off to the footy together, father and son. The next, we're skidding off the road, my knuckles are turning white on the steering wheel, I'm fearing the worst. There's nothing I can do. I've lost control of the car from the left-hand lane, we've gone careering exactly where we cannot afford to go—further left. We mount the kerb and hit a telegraph pole.

By the time I stumble out of the wreckage, I'm in shock. Josh is still sitting in the car. Apart from a small scrape on Josh's arm, neither of us have a scratch. The police arrive. They tell me the car is so badly damaged they expected to be retrieving bodies from the vehicle. I've thought about this event many times. Someone or something was looking after us that day.

I've asked Josh a number of times if I was driving over the limit. If I was, he would tell me so in no uncertain terms. I know I wasn't speeding, but when the police got an eye witness to confirm I was under the 70 kilometre per hour speed limit, that eased my conscience no end. (But it's still a memory that makes me feel sick to the pit of my stomach when I think about it, which I still do from time to time.)

The car is a mess, but we escape with our lives. I never want this kind of experience again. By the time Louise arrives at the scene I am manic. The shock of the accident has thrown me into a tailspin. An ambulance takes us to a local hospital, where we're assessed for injuries, x-rayed from head to toe and given the all clear. Practically as soon as we've walked into the hospital, we're walking out again. The car is a write-off, so badly damaged it ends up on the back of a tow truck. Louise's sister, Christine, arrives and drives us all back home. The mania is under control for now so there's no trouble.

Back home, I try to relax with a nice hot bath. I settle down in front of the TV to watch the game I was supposed to be calling. The Roosters against the Dragons is a traditional clash on a very important day for all Australians and New Zealanders. I try to calm down, enjoy what is about to unfold on the tube. The shock of the accident, though, just the raw realisation that my son and I were almost killed, starts really kicking in.

Some six hours after the accident, during halftime in the game, I'm fully psychotic. Louise thinks I might cause a problem or two. She calls the police. Fair enough: I have a little history.

19 Take care you don't drown in self-pity

When I was suffering, I think I wanted others to share my suffering. So they knew what I was going through. Perhaps so I got sympathy; so I was noticed. But it's a human frailty that I'm banishing from my life. I don't want your sympathy any more; I want to give you mine. When I feel empowered and on top of the world, I want everyone to feel as good as I do. I want to keep the positive emotions while eliminating the negative.

When I realised this, something clicked—loudly. My battles have toughened me up and opened my eyes. I used to *act* resilient and open-minded, but now I *feel* it. We have to be honest about our weaknesses and if anything is to be gained from them.

Something is keeping me on this spiritual path. Something is telling me this is right and real. I am interested in what that something is. I'm determined to stick with these spiritual explorations and see where they lead. I know I'll swerve off course. I know I'll make wrong turns, let some people down, let myself down. But at the end of every experience, whether enlightened or doomed or somewhere in between, I'll remember to be kind to myself. I'll never expect myself or anyone else to be perfect.

We all have imperfections. We've all lost a few teeth along the way. Why? Because we are human beings. I might completely fall off the road if mania revisits. Will this book make a positive difference to me or anyone else? I hope so . . . Maybe you're thinking of what Groucho Marx said of an acquaintance's book: 'From the moment I picked up your book until I laid it down, I was convulsed with laughter. Some day, I intend reading it.' Maybe that's you, but it doesn't matter. All anyone can do is try. Instead of us being physical human beings undergoing a brief spiritual experience, I'm starting to believe we're actually spiritual beings having a brief human experience.

How did I reach these realisations? *The Seat of the Soul* by Gary Zukav tweaked my perceptions up another few notches. It's a New York Times #1 bestseller full of transfixing passages:

> We are evolving from five-sensory humans into multisensory humans. The perceptions of the multisensory human extend beyond physical reality to the larger dynamical systems of which our physical reality is a part. We are evolving from a species that pursues external power into a species that pursues authentic power. Authentic power has its roots in the deepest source of our being. An authentically empowered person is incapable of making anyone or anything a victim. An authentically empowered person is one who is so strong, so empowered, that the idea of using force against another is not a part of his or her consciousness.

That blows me away.

20 Authenticity takes you places

What I've learned is that every time we're prepared to be authentic, we make a difference—to ourselves and to those around us. Something inside is set free. Often we're afraid of baring our souls, but as the famous baseball player Babe Ruth advised: 'Never let the fear of striking out stand in your way.'

Rugby league great Andrew Johns had the courage to reveal his long-term battle with depression in an interview with Phil Gould on the Nine Network's *The Footy Show* in 2007. Watching Andrew discuss his internal battles in front of a TV audience of millions was compelling viewing. No-one thought less of him. Indeed, and importantly, and there's a strong message in this: he went up in most people's estimation. People appreciate honesty, whether it's delivered in front of a TV camera or across the kitchen table.

Andrew had always been a bit of a wild character and now we knew why. He's the best rugby league player I've ever seen. He did things on a footy field that others can only dream of. I watched almost every on-field move while working for the ABC in Newcastle. He played his entire career with the Knights and I got to know him pretty well through interviews and a bit of social interaction.

I could see from early on that he was a complex character. Some days, he would be happy-go-lucky, laughing it up and joking round. Other days, he would be intense and withdrawn. It took me a while to get a handle on that. I remember a conversation with Andrew at Sydney Airport, not long after I'd been diagnosed with bipolar. Andrew told me about his own highs and lows and I remember thinking at the time that Andrew must also be bipolar.

His focus these days is on relaxing. He lives on the northern beaches of Sydney, away from Newcastle, where he's too much of a famous figure to be left alone.

'The most important thing for me these days, to manage the highs and lows of bipolar, is the ocean,' he says. 'Getting in the surf and riding waves, sometimes for most of the day, centres and grounds me.

'Those two things are so critical with an illness like bipolar disorder. Just to get out there in the ocean is complete freedom to me. It doesn't matter, to the bloke surfing the same break, if it's Andrew Johns or whoever surfing with him; we're just out there getting waves together. We're there for the same reasons: to relax, escape and rejuvenate. It's fantastic.

'My old coach at the Newcastle Knights, Michael Hagan, got me into an alternative therapy called reiki,' Andrew tells me. 'It's very different and it's surprised me how beneficial it's been. I feel absolutely relaxed, with the weight of the world lifted off my shoulders. This calm, relaxed state lasts for two or three days after a session. All of that, and the therapist doesn't even lay a hand on me. That's pretty wild, if you ask me.

'I take fish-oil capsules, Omega 3, every day, as well as my prescribed medication of Epilim every morning and night. Taking my medication is just part of my daily routine now. When I get out of bed and brush my teeth, I take my morning dose. The last thing before going to bed at night, I take the other dose. It's become habit. No dramas, it's just very important I keep that up.

'The other thing I need is regular sleep. Without a good night's sleep I become frayed around the edges, which is when I can quickly become manic. A good sleep is critical to me staying balanced and well. Of all these things, though, probably the most important, apart from medication, is routine. I really need routine. If I don't know what I'm doing for the next three or four days, my mind begins to wander . . . For example Monday: Football coverage with Channel Nine. Tuesday: Take my son Samuel to school, have a surf. Wednesday: Exercise session. Thursday: meeting with Channel Nine for *The Footy Show*. Friday: Golf, footy commentary for Channel Nine that night. And then it starts all over again. That's just a rough plan but they're the certainties I need. I'm very conscious of having routines and sticking to them.

'My mates know me very well, too, and look out for me. They know the danger signs when I start getting a little high. It's a quiet tap on the shoulder from them and a word of advice: "Andrew, slow down, relax; you're running high." I'm lucky to have them around me and, these days, I actually do listen to them. We all learn our lessons, some of us more slowly than others.'

21 What works for Wally Lewis

Wally opened up about his battle with depression in another widely watched TV interview. He became suicidal at his lowest point, too. Every man in Australia fell off his chair, thinking: 'Wally Lewis? *The* Wally Lewis?' Wally battled epilepsy for more than 25 years before having it operated on. He suffered a fit on live TV, the ultimate disaster in his field.

I can imagine it would be awkward enough on live radio, let alone the most widely watched sports report in Queensland. Clinical depression followed as sure as night follows day: again, this was *the* Wally Lewis, former captain of the Australian rugby league team. One of the most unbreakable sportsmen to have represented his nation. He had the entire state of NSW booing him in Origin matches in Sydney, throwing beer cans at him, offering every insult under the sun, and he did not bat an eyelid.

Wally was as mentally tough as a man can get—but even he was floored by depression. See? It really can happen to anyone. See? No reason to be ashamed. So much praise is thrown Wally's way and he deserves the lot of it. He was a great leader. My initial view of him, from a distance, was that he was arrogant, but I had him oh-so wrong. He's humble and in telling his story he's had an impact on many lives.

After his operation for epilepsy, the doctor ordered complete rest for more than seven months. That's when Wally slid into clinical depression. He thanks his family and in particular his wife, Jenny, for supporting him during that time. He began a course of antidepressant medication, which he takes to this day. He came up to me a while ago, after an NRL game at the new stadium in Melbourne, and asked how I was travelling.

My answer was that I had good days and bad. He said he was the same. An important part of his recovery has been banning the booze. 'I have not touched any alcohol for nearly twenty years,' he says. 'I gave it up completely after a binge drinking session one night with a couple of my old teammates from the Broncos, Allan Langer and Kevin Walters. I wasn't going to drink but they basically said come on, Wally, let's all have a drink for old time's sake. I relented but that's been my only relapse on the grog in two decades. I don't miss it—and I certainly don't miss the hangovers.

'My health is good these days and I intend to keep it that way by living well with family and friends close by. I love a game of golf, although I haven't played much lately. The Jack Newton Celebrity Classic has been a favourite of mine every year. But the most important thing of all is just relaxing. Having a conversation with my mates, taking it easy. I never used to do that enough. So much of my life, up until my seizures and operation for epilepsy, had been spent under extreme pressure. That wasn't healthy, as I found out. My family has been unbelievable. I'm almost certain that I could not have done it without them. I don't know how I would have reacted if the roles had been reversed. The love and support I am given is amazing and so important.'

22 Mark Gable's fable

Few people know that the lead singer of the Choirboys has also fought the demons. I grew up listening to this band. They were the quintessential Australian rock'n'rollers: 'Run to Paradise' is a well-known anthem to anyone who was out and about in the 1980s. Mark is a charismatic figure as lead singer. It shocked me to learn he was slugged with clinical depression. Rock stars, with all the bravado they need to get up on stage, are one of those stereotyped groups you think of as being untouchable.

I first met Mark at a *beyondblue* function for the Canterbury–Bankstown rugby league club in Sydney. We had a connection straight away and sat together over lunch with Mark's partner, the singer-songwriter Melinda Schneider. Before meeting Mark, I'd had no idea about his depression. He was fantastically honest about it. At a later date, when he came to Newcastle to promote the Choirboys' 30th anniversary tour, we spoke at length in the ABC studio, off-air, before our formal interview started for the listeners. I told Mark I was really wrestling the black dog again. He was so supportive. Twenty-four hours later, he sent me a text to see how I was going. That made my day. He cheered me up simply by showing he cared.

Mark's behavioural changes have been significant. A rock'n'roll lifestyle doesn't exactly complement a mental health problem. Eliminating alcohol has been a big part of his recovery, too.

'I don't drink at all,' Mark says. 'I haven't touched it in six years. Of course, for much of the time I was with the Choirboys, alcohol was a huge part of the scene and I certainly got stuck into it. I've given up caffeine, too.

'I started drinking green tea but became quite addicted to that. I was drinking seven to eight cups per day because I was told it was good for me. But I found out green tea has caffeine, so I hadn't actually given it up at all. I had to start all over again, this time kicking my green-tea addiction. I don't touch soft drink. My drinks of choice are water and peppermint tea—only.

'As far as food goes, I have porridge with soy or rice milk. I've given up processed sugar, which I think is really important. I felt awful when I first gave it up. For two weeks, I was run-down, had no energy—but after that my energy increased and went higher than it had been in a long time. I gave up processed foods. These days I'm on a low GI diet—it's basically a diet for diabetics, with a little more latitude.

'I've done kinesiology. CBT has been important: cognitive behavioural therapy. I was pretty messed up when I tried it, having just had my first very bad bout of depression. I was going through a rough relationship break-up and was drinking heavily. I went through a period of four to five years of heavy drinking, binge drinking four or five days a week. I was 44 when I really got stuck into the drink. Then came the depression, when all I wanted to do was have another drink, which led to an even bigger second depression. I gave up alcohol by just waking up one day saying, "No more." I tried professional counselling, which I found to be very helpful. Obviously, nothing beats the support of friends and family.

'My environment is also very important and I believe it is for everyone. The people you associate with can determine your whole lifestyle. A lot of people I used to associate with have dropped off because I've stopped drinking. I'm fine with that. I'm no longer part of that scene and as for those past associations, I guess it wasn't meant to be. I know a lot of people enjoy yoga but I don't like it. My yoga, my experience of being in the moment, is walking. I find it very relaxing. It clears my mind. I'm very aware of my thoughts and body when I'm walking.'

23 How Garry McDonald takes the edge off his anxiety

Actor Garry McDonald has been front and centre in two of the finest comedy programs in the history of Australian TV: *The Norman Gunston Show* and *Mother and Son*. He's another to have been struck by anxiety and depression. The trigger for Garry was the pressure of writing and producing his weekly comedy program for our TV screens. He cracked, but he's another Australian male who has turned a harrowing part of his life into a positive through his role as a board director for *beyondblue*. He's touched a lot of people: more than 3000 people in one go, for example. I know because I was right there with him . . .

It was at a conference called Happiness and its Causes. The venue was the Sydney Convention and Exhibition Centre at Darling Harbour. Garry and I were asked to speak about our personal experiences with depression. We were to be interviewed on stage by Leonie Young, who at the time was the chief executive officer of *beyondblue*. We got to the Convention Centre and I was stunned—3500 people were crammed inside. It's an enormous place, a terrific arena, and it was practically a sell-out. It was going to be the biggest crowd I'd ever spoken in front of, but I wasn't nervous. I knew what I wanted to say—and Garry was such a pro that we could barely go wrong. Still, it was a *little* daunting because the first speaker on the day, the keynote speaker and the reason there were so many people there at 9 a.m., was His Holiness the Dalai Lama.

To be in the same room and hear such a revered man was an experience in itself. I hung on his every word. He went over all the themes and messages he's written and talked about: compassion, understanding, peace, the importance of meditation and having self-discipline, contentment. The biggest message was that all these skills could be learned. People shifted forward in their seats when they heard that, including me. It's what we all wanted to know: we *can* do it.

People assume you either have serenity or you don't. His Holiness was saying if you have it, hang on to it for dear sweet life. If you don't, reach out and grab it because *everyone* can if they know where to look and if they dedicate themselves to the search. Even if we fall a little—or a lot—short of his rarefied level of contentment, we'll still be better off than we are now.

You could have heard a pin drop during a one-hour talk that floated over us for what felt like five minutes. He was fantastic, quietly spoken as you'd imagine, with a quirky little sense of humour. He kept coming up with lines that made himself laugh. He'd giggle and smile like a cheeky little boy and then 3500 people would start giggling with him. He just had a wonderful way. He looked as if he was enjoying the experience himself, and that rubbed off on the people listening. Another subtle lesson.

After the Dalai Lama, there was a discussion to be hosted by Geraldine Doogue from the ABC's *Compass* program. The comedian Magda Szubanski was on the panel, so was Professor Gordon Parker from the Black Dog Institute. Garry and I were supposed to be on stage at 11.30 a.m. But the guy who was scheduled before us, something went wrong with his Power-Point presentation—don't ask me what—but the long and short of it was that his technology failed him at the last minute. His whole presentation relied on the PowerPoint component, so he was a goner.

Garry and I got a tap on the shoulder: change of plans, you two are on next. They whisked us out the back, down the side of the stage, through a couple of doors, and through an underground maze of corridors inside the Convention Centre. We got wired up with our little Madonna microphones, those ones you can hardly see, we trotted onto the stage—and it was just a great experience. We seemed to be received warmly enough even though I could imagine people thinking: Well, that Craig Hamilton ain't no Dalai Lama.

Leonie interviewed us, walking (and talking) us through our stories. I think we were up there for about 45 minutes. Garry and I bounced off each other pretty well, we got a few laughs. It was thoroughly enjoyable and privilege being on stage with someone of his calibre. I relished every minute of it. Best of all, though, and the thing that has made me laugh ever since, is that Garry and I can spend the rest of our lives telling people about the time we had the Dalai Lama as our warm-up act.

Norman Gunston was a truly brilliant comedy creation. I remember watching Garry/Norman interview Muhammad Ali and Paul McCartney: two of the funniest things I have ever seen in my life. His other brilliant show was *Mother and Son* with Ruth Cracknell. So I knew he was a versatile actor.

What I didn't know was he also suffered very serious depression and anxiety, enough for him to contemplate ending it all, too. It came to a head for Garry when he tried to resurrect *The Norman Gunston Show* for prime-time TV. A week or two before the show was due to go to air, one of the producers walked away. The responsibility of putting the show together was almost single-handedly Garry's, and it critically affected his health. A major breakdown was the inevitable result. Garry has spoken many times on TV and in public about his battle with anxiety and depression.

In a *beyondblue* interview he said:

> My first experience with anxiety was straight after smoking marijuana and hashish. It frightened me. I didn't touch it again for twenty years. I tried it again and had yet another experience with dreadful anxiety. I didn't get depressed until twenty years later—everything was going wrong with the TV show. I got blind drunk with the executive producer and the channel heavyweights of the day, which didn't help one bit. I had major depression by this stage and was put on antidepressant medication. What really worked for me was cognitive behavioural therapy. I did a little bit of talking about the situation, but not too much.
>
> The part I held on to was the negative thoughts in my head. I had to challenge those thoughts. What proof was there about them being right? Whatever the negative thought was, my cognitive behaviour therapy told me to challenge that thought. Where's the proof? I also meditate twice a day. I find meditation fantastic—it's a skill that can be learned and practised anywhere from your own house to a hotel room, wherever you happen to be. It makes me feel like I can deal with any situation. Not always, or probably not as often as I should, I go for a walk. I'd recommend a daily walk to anyone. It always starts my day well, really lifts my spirits.

That's two walkers—Garry and Mark. I used to think only John Howard did it. I'll be joining in soon enough.

24 Jessica Rowe—a real inspiration

Women are not immune to these issues. They may not have caves to retreat to like us bone-headed men; they may not go and hide under a rock when there's a personal issue to confront, but lows can hit them just as hard. Postnatal depression can come as a huge shock. Motherhood is supposed to be so enriching. Jessica Rowe is a well-known Australian journalist and TV presenter who speaks from the heart about her postnatal depression following the birth of her first daughter, Allegra. A more delightful person than Jessica you're unlikely to meet. Allegra now has a little sister, Giselle.

The twist to the tale is that Jessica's mother, Penelope, is bipolar. She's lived with it for nearly 50 years but was only diagnosed in her early 30s. Jessica, the eldest of Penelope's three daughters, whom she raised as a single mother, saw the effects of bipolar from close range. Her mum was a frequent visitor to psychiatric hospitals and Jessica recalls how powerless she felt during Penelope's depressions. Jessica's tale is the remarkable life story of a remarkable woman. Through her own experiences, and from seeing Penelope's battles from the closest possible range—under the same roof—Jessica has intimate knowledge of what she so rightly calls an unpredictable enemy. 'When I had Allegra,

I was desperate to be a mum, busting to be a mum,' she says. 'I went through IVF and luckily on our third attempt, I became pregnant. I was like, "This is fantastic, all my dreams are coming true."

'Unfortunately, it wasn't as wonderful as I'd hoped at the start. I had postnatal depression, like one in seven mums do. (I'm sure the real number is probably higher.) It was a really tough time. I remember going to my first mother's group, and I'd never felt so alone and isolated. It really surprised me because I think sometimes, as women, we can be one another's greatest supporters, but we can also be one another's worst enemies when we're not honest with each other.

'I remember other new mums saying, "Oh, isn't this the happiest you've ever been? Doesn't this just get better and better!" And I was thinking to myself, No! That actually isn't how I'm feeling at all! But I didn't have the courage or the confidence to say that. Over time I began to tell myself, "I know I'm not the only one who's struggling." I was really yearning for honest, open conversation.'

Ongoing conversation between men, women, all of us, is where answers will come from. One of the things that resonated with me in speaking to Andrew, Wally and Mark in particular was the issue of alcohol. When battling the highs and lows of bipolar disorder I have had my own challenges. The most important lesson for me to learn through all this was that alcohol was not the answer to any problem I had.

25 The thing about alcohol

Among the men I've spoken to for this book, banishing alcohol has obviously been a major theme. I really do understand the need to ditch it. It can be hard because, under the rules and regulations of blokedom, having a beer is one of our rites. It's so Australian. If you're catching up with a mate, you go have a beer. If there's a celebration, anything from a 21st birthday to New Year's Eve to the Melbourne Cup, everyone gets on it. I used to imbibe as enthusiastically as the next bloke, and more enthusiastically than the bloke next to him. I used to binge drink to excess, but not any more.

My alcohol intake these days is the bare minimum. It's just no good for me. It does not mix well with my medications (or any medications) but, more to the point, I don't *need* it. I've grown out of it. Think of the people most in tune with themselves, those who are the happiest and most content and comfortable in their own skins, and they're not the ones who need half-a-dozen schooners to function in a social situation.

The legendary rugby league coach Wayne Bennett, who wrote the foreword to my first book, has helped point me in the right direction. He was in Newcastle for a charity fundraiser in early 2011 and my job on the night was to MC the event and interview Wayne. We sat together and it was a great experience because I really enjoy his company. He talks a lot more freely socially than he does in a typical media interview! He is actually a very funny bloke and loves a good laugh.

Wayne, as usual, was drinking water and an occasional orange juice. I asked him at what age he gave up alcohol. His reply nearly floored me. Wayne said he'd never had an alcoholic drink in his life—not one. I'd read his books and seen the wonderful TV program *Australian Story* that featured Wayne and his family. I knew his childhood was tough, as he'd grown up with an alcoholic father who caused plenty of problems at home. When he was fourteen, Wayne gave a commitment to his mother that he would never drink. And he never has.

I'm moving closer all the time to becoming a complete non-drinker. I've gradually consumed less and less to the point where the very most I'll have in one day is two light beers, or a glass of wine, when we go out to dinner. That's the very upper limit. More often than not, I'll have an orange juice or soda water with lime and lemon and feel like a million bucks. I'm not an absolute teetotaller but if somebody told me I had to completely abstain from tomorrow, never touching another drop, I would not care less.

Alcohol clouds my judgement. It shuts down clear thinking, harms my physical wellbeing and takes me away from the more spiritual path I'm convinced is doing me good. And anyway, I'm just over it and no longer feel the urge. I can be sitting at a table with a group of ten people, everyone else having seven or eight beers each over the course of a night. I can very happily sit there nursing my soda water and juice without feeling out of place. That's just my choice these days.

Bipolar comes with its own depressant. I don't need a top-up, thanks very much.

I don't miss out on any part of the conversation. I can still engage with everyone. If it's a night function and the evening lingers, I end up making more sense than anyone! And I can get in my car and drive home with a clear conscience. In my view, alcohol is the most damaging drug in Australia. Alcohol is routinely a contributing factor or the sole cause of deaths on the road, domestic violence, street violence, unsociable behaviour, family breakdown, financial hardship, assault, time lost in the workplace, road accidents, life-threatening illnesses . . . the list goes on and on.

I almost want to be breath-tested after a night out so I can bask in the glory of my zero reading. I'm zero on the RBT and zero on my psychiatrist Dr Weiss's scale of minus- to plus-five. Perfect. Case in point: I attended a Hawthorn Club lunch in Newcastle before the Rugby World Cup where Australia's coach Robbie Deans was the guest speaker. I drank my soda water and had a great time. The blokes at my table could not have cared less. That's because they were real mates. If a group of drinkers are uneasy about having me around, well, whose problem is that?

The most important thing is how I feel about myself. In times of trouble, I highly recommend looking seriously at the amount of alcohol you're pouring into your system. I'm acutely aware that this lifestyle choice isn't for everyone, so there will be no crusade on it from me. Some of my best mates have always enjoyed alcohol in moderation and have it completely under control.

A chilled glass of white wine at the end of a summer's day probably has a bit going for it. But the stance I've taken has made me feel ten years younger. Alcohol, hangovers—I'm glad to have left them behind. I shall continue drinking only from the fountain of rediscovered youth. However, I have also discovered that staying away from the booze and taking better care of myself is no guarantee that bipolar disorder won't affect my life again.

26 Don't define yourself by your condition

It's liberating when you can recognise honestly where you're at. It mightn't be easy, but it's worth all the discomfort. When I can be open I learn things too. I discover that I'm not alone, that by speaking out we can help each other. Here's one letter I received that touched a chord:

> I have a current diagnosis of schizoaffective disorder, a cross between bipolar and schizophrenia. I cope very well now, working full-time, balancing family and work life. I do look after myself with a healthy diet, plenty of exercise and adequate sleep. However, I have a tendency to work too many hours, getting carried away with my own magnificence—you know the story.
>
> My initial story is a horrific nightmare—similar in many ways to yours. However I have had plenty of time to get used to living with mental health issues, and refuse to become a victim to them. Out of the years has grown an understanding and acceptance. Perhaps most importantly, I have learned to be assertive and recognise my own limitations. I am able to say 'no' and feel good about that. I know that I have to protect my own health in the interests of myself and my family.
>
> I battle with frequent bouts of depression. However, although it is really awful and black, I know that there is light at the end of the tunnel. I try to view it as having the same path (although obviously with more severity) as a common cold. It will run its course, I will get

better, but at some stage I will have another bout. I feel acceptance is vital. One can do everything possible to help oneself, but fighting and non-acceptance only add to the anxiety and stress levels.

My psychotic episodes are thankfully far less frequent, and I find them terrifying. I have never got beyond that. It is the fear of losing control of my mind and my life. I haven't been manic for ten years, although I still have to watch myself and recognise the risk factors. I am not immune from it happening again.

One of the issues that I have constantly battled with is 'coming out'. I experienced numerous incidents in the early years of being undermined, undervalued and just plain not taken seriously because of my mental health issues. 'Yes, well, we all know about her, etc, etc.'

As the years have gone by, I constantly question how much information it is safe to reveal, especially in the workplace. I value my increased ability to support and empathise with others. Yet I am only too aware that some people will use my history to undermine me. I have spoken at a few meetings, but more commonly on a much smaller scale. I have been able to greatly increase the understanding of some individuals on mental health issues and thus their ability to support others. Yet I have also found there can be a high price to pay for speaking out. It's a juggling act and one that there are no clear answers for.

I wholeheartedly agree that raising awareness doesn't only stem from talking to a packed-out conference hall of 300 people. It can be as simple as sharing a quiet word with someone who is still coming to terms with their diagnosis. Reading about being carried away with your own magnificence—that brought a smile to my face. And it reminds me of Oscar Wilde: 'I am so clever that sometimes I don't understand a single word of what I am saying!'

So how do you move on when you know there are some big battles ahead? There was a time when I thought I had the illness beat. How wrong I was. I gave up yoga. I stopped taking my medication. I thought the bipolar was gone, that it was just a temporary aberration in my life. I'd beaten it! Normal transmission had been resumed. The dangers associated with that kind of smug thinking are immense.

I found out in the most brutal fashion when depression knocked me out for nine months. I had three psychotic episodes in four years, all because I was complacent. I still needed medication, daily, without fail. It's now been a year without a manic episode.

> I'm managing my illness instead of letting it manage me.

Does that just mean I'm due for another? Is another blow-up just around the corner? Reading that someone has gone ten years without an episode is comforting, but I know enough to understand it'll probably happen again. I'm not going to live in fear of it. As long as I do everything in my power to stay medicated and healthy, there's nothing more I can hope for. I will simply do my best day after day and hope the days become incident-free for months and years on end. The rest is in the lap of the gods. I sleep easy at night. I'm managing my illness instead of letting it manage me.

Never define yourself by your condition. I'm a husband, father and sports commentator. I just happen to have bipolar. I have an illness but the illness isn't who I am. I go about my business, and go about my life, just the same as everyone else. The secret is about being in it for the whole journey, the good bits and the seriously hard bits.

Back to hospital

ANZAC DAY 2007 (continued): The constabulary arrive and sit in our lounge room, the football commentary a bizarre backdrop to our fifteen-minute conversation. The discussion is cool and calm. I agree to be taken to James Fletcher Hospital. The kite starts coming down. I'm assessed and voluntarily admitted. En route to the ward I run into my old mate Martin Drinkwater. Martin is the mental health nurse who treated me with great compassion and care when I had my first psychotic episode.

Martin works in the Waratah wing, the maximum security section of James Fletcher. He's just finishing his shift when he sees me being wheeled through the hospital on a mobile bed. He smiles and says: 'Think you're God again, mate?' I have a chuckle, give him a thumbs up and say: 'Nah, mate. I'm Craig this time.' I like it when people refuse to skirt around the issue. He says he's very pleased to hear it—and leaves for the day.

The more Martin Drinkwaters in this world, the better. And sure enough, after being admitted to the main lockdown ward in the hospital the first four people I meet are named Jesus. A dilemma easily over-come, however: 'OK,' says one, 'I'll be Jesus number 1, you can be Jesus number 2 . . .' and so on. Problem solved.

I am transferred to the Lindgard Private Hospital at Merewether and spend two weeks coming down from the high. It's great to get visitors at

Lindgard . . . people are slowly but surely getting used to walking into a psychiatric ward without thinking twice.

A major depression turns up to wipe me off my feet. I've been expecting it. Lows invariably follow highs or maybe the expectation has become a self-fulfilling prophecy. This one fails to disappoint. We take a family holiday to Fiji for five days in the mistaken belief that lying in the sun will help. The stranger inside is taking hold again, moving in, getting awfully comfortable, sneering at me from the corners of my mind.

I take my medication: 50 milligrams of an antidepressant called Pristiq. It does nothing. The doctors give me approval to take 100 milligrams a day. An entire month passes before I start to improve. Four Sundays come and go without me hosting 'Grandstand' on the ABC. No travelling to country NSW with David Morrow and Warren Ryan. I don't see them—or anyone—for the longest time. I may as well have fallen off the face of the Earth.

I'm prescribed the antipsychotic and mood stabiliser Zyprexa, which is also useful for treating depression. I'm sleeping a lot, but there's only one thing that really eases the pain, albeit fleetingly. For months I do this, dragging myself to the beach in the middle of winter. No-one else is in the water. The beach is deserted. The ocean is frigid at about fifteen degrees. I dive in and while I'm below the surface, out of sight and mind of the rest of the world, I do the only thing I can think of to release the frustration and tension building within: I scream at the top of my lungs.

Gradually the depression lifts again and life returns to normality. I feel well and go back to work. Once again I am blessed to return to a workplace that does not discriminate against people with a diagnosed mental illness. The ABC is truly a world-class employer.

27 Why support at work is critical

The best and most understanding boss wants to know why you're early for work instead of being at home with your family. Wants to know why you haven't taken a lunch break, why you're eating in front of your computer and why you're still at your desk an hour and a half after finishing time. These are not meaningless, petty questions but major psychological enquiries: *why* are you still here when you don't have to be?

The best and most understanding boss wants you fit, well, relaxed and working at a premium level during regular working hours, but understands you need downtime when you do not have to give the office, or anyone in it (including the head honcho), any mind. The most clued-up boss knows that longer hours do not equate to higher productivity.

I thought bipolar disorder would spell the end of my career as a radio broadcaster for the ABC. I would be stamped too much of a risk for live-to-air work, which would mean I'd be unable to work at all. I would be shattered beyond belief when I was given the news but, even worse, I would be able to understand their position.

The ABC is built upon respect and professionalism. No-one at head office would feel particularly good about kicking me to the kerb, but I felt sure they would have to. What if Jesus Christ reared his head during Sunday afternoon football? What if I lost the plot in an interview? *I'm with Newcastle coach Wayne Bennett— and Wayne, do you realise Nelson Mandela will be joining us soon? Are you aware, Wayne, that I have many spiritual powers?* The mere risk of it was unacceptable. What if St Francis of Assisi decided to save all the souls in the Newcastle Knights' dressing room? Then what? I'd be sacked before I got back to my car. My life would amount to sitting around all day with a blanket on my lap, staring out the window, listening to ABC radio, racked with jealousy of whoever had taken my place. Back to the coalmines for me, once I got that blanket off my lap. Or, more likely, off to grow chokoes for a living. Nothing wrong with the mines—or growing chokoes for that matter—but I was just getting revved up in a job I loved.

> 'A person is a success if he gets up in the morning and goes to bed at night and in between does what he wants to do.'
>
> Bob Dylan

How I underestimated my employers. From day one, when the ABC found out I wouldn't be at the Olympics and might be unpredictable for some time to come, it has accommodated every new need that has arisen, including time off at the last moment. I have never been made to feel guilty. I've never picked up the most remote vibe that I have been letting anyone down or becoming a burden. The opposite has been true. It is such a caring and supportive atmosphere and proves what can be done when the employer's attitude is right. The message has been this from the outset: we're on your side, Craig. We're here to help.

I can't emphasise enough the positive affect of emotional support on an employee with depression. It makes me want to pay the ABC back in spades for the rest of my career. Even after the initial reassurances, I still feared it might go pear-shaped. That just one on-air incident would make the situation untenable. Rightly or wrongly, fact or fiction, it felt like I might be on probation. But when pear-shaped did come, a few times over, such as my lacklustre performance at Parramatta Stadium and my early-morning withdrawal from commitments the following day, thankfully I was far from a microphone when I hit full swing and the ABC was professional enough to quickly arrange cover in Canberra, where I was supposed to be the next day.

The ABC bosses understand the cyclical nature of the illness. There will be times, even long times, when I am unavailable—it's just a fact. But there are also long periods without incident. Good management, and good luck, has averted disaster. Just because someone has bipolar disorder, just because anyone out there has a mental illness, it doesn't mean we can't be terrific employees. You don't have to lock us in the cupboard. Live radio is probably the least suitable profession for the psychologically volatile but if I've been able to keep going, I reckon most other jobs out there are eminently do-able. I don't mean in terms of just plodding through. I feel like I'm thriving simply from knowing my employer supports me. A great job can still be done. I feel I have the ABC's trust and that I've earned it. Andrew Johns and Wally Lewis are on live TV. No problems for them, either.

> Just because someone has bipolar disorder, just
> because anyone out there has a mental illness, it
> doesn't mean we can't be terrific employees.

For everything I've said about keeping the work–life balance in check, I'm not downplaying the importance of work at all. It's still enormously important to wellbeing in terms of independence, both emotionally and financially, and personal satisfaction.

I maintain it shouldn't be allowed to dominate our lives, but it should still be tackled with gusto at the appropriate times.

An old truism: the trick is to find a job that doesn't feel like work. Something that you're interested in and passionate about anyway. Something you enjoy so much that you arrive at the end of an eight-hour shift and think, where did the time go? If I wasn't calling the NRL, I'd be watching and listening to it anyway. I want to work the house down during the hours I'm allotted, but on my days off and before and after my shifts, I keep myself and my work fresh by blocking it out. Knowing when to switch off is as important as when to switch on and rip in.

There's scope for bosses to manage mental illness. I was at the mercy of the ABC, but it's been twelve years since the great train robbery of my senses at Broadmeadow, and it looks like we're going to stick. The key is being ahead of the game, knowing when there might be trouble on the horizon, and letting people know. Again, honesty is paramount. I want to keep my bosses informed. They don't want to be guessing any more than I do. I have to recognise the warning signs—and heed them.

The human temptation and my residual blokedom is to convince myself everything will be OK, to pretend there isn't any drama, that I'm completely on top of it. But it's vital to be proactive. Even though the damage was limited, I wasn't proactive enough that night at Parramatta Stadium. I'll be more honest with Steve Mortimer next time. Was I OK? Not really. I might not have known what was brewing, but I knew it was unusual for me to be so uninterested in our call and in the game itself. I want to nip episodes like that in the bud.

The setbacks and missed opportunities along the way have been frustrating, there's no denying that. Back in 2000, I couldn't go back to work until I was cleared by a Commonwealth-appointed psychiatrist. The first four or five times, he said no, application rejected: I still wasn't right. From when I was hospitalised, it took two months to get the all-clear. That might not sound like long, all things considered, but it felt interminable.

I was in hospital for twelve days, was forced to take those two months off work and then came the gradual return of assured-ness behind the microphone. It wasn't as confronting as being told: Here you go, mate, there's the microphone, go get 'em. No pressure was placed on me. The ABC said it would keep an eye on me, ease me back in, let me do it at whatever pace I felt comfortable with.

A job well done puts a spring in my step. It's genuine happi-ness and an ideal adrenaline buzz when a call has gone well and I'm driving back on the freeway from Sydney to Newcastle, music blaring. It proves work does have sizeable benefits to your psyche when it's approached the right way, as a part of life but not the dominant force. Like Mark Gable says, environment is crucial: I cannot overstate the importance of surrounding yourself with positive people. The ABC is wall-to-wall with broadcasters who make me aspire to be as good as I can in this profession. It doesn't matter what field you're in, you can aim to be fantastic at it. You're a janitor? You can be the greatest janitor who ever lived.

> I cannot overstate the importance of surrounding yourself with positive people.

The higher the levels of dedication and professionalism among your colleagues, the better your chances of success. I do have tremendous respect for sports commentators outside the ABC. Channel Nine's Ray Warren is passionate and accurate. Ray Hadley is an outstanding commentator and broadcaster for 2GB whose versatility is tremendous. But I believe the ABC has Australia's premier sports callers, with icons such as Jim Maxwell, Warren Ryan, Peter Wilkins and David Morrow.

Jim Maxwell: just the familiarity to Australians of that voice in summer . . . he took the chair from Alan McGilvray as the ABC's chief cricket commentator back in 1985 when Alan broadcast his last Test match at the famous Sydney Cricket Ground. Jim has gone on to call a record number of Tests and one-day internationals. He's unfailingly consistent. A day of Test cricket can be seven hours and patience is a necessity: Jim can be understated, which suits cricket, or he can be conversational, which is important when there are so many lulls between deliveries and overs.

Peter Wilkins has also been there for me. We don't see much of each other these days as our working lives have changed direction, but he has offered me support during the tough times. He is also very good for a laugh, and that's important.

In rugby league, Warren Ryan has his critics, no doubt about it. He rubs plenty of people the wrong way because he speaks his mind. Well, all I'll say in response is that the truth sometimes hurts. 'Wok' is rugby league through and through, and underneath the tough exterior is a heart of gold. Believe me, I've seen it. Wok has a fine-tuned, dry sense of humour. His favourite quote is this, from Winston Churchill: 'Here's a man who, if he tripped over the truth, would quickly get to his feet and move on as though nothing had happened.' His passion for rugby league knows no bounds. At the end of an NRL season, I'm usually pretty tired and ready for a break. A few years ago, we'd just taken our headsets off in the commentary box after the grand final. I was stuffed, thinking: Thank goodness that's over, I really need a break. Warren said: 'Jeez, I wish it was on again next week!'

Even Wok's staunchest critics must acknowledge his influence on how the game is played and coached today. He's the best analyst in the game. NRL coaches still seek his views and opinions on their teams and opposition. Phil Gould coached two sides to premiership wins, and is NSW's most successful State of

Origin coach. In his autobiography, Phil writes that as far as he's concerned, there's only been one real Supercoach. Not Wayne Bennett; not Jack Gibson: Warren Ryan.

I've been on the end of Wok's gruff style and it's left me momentarily questioning his methods. One day at Sydney's Kogarah Oval we were getting ready to broadcast a St George game, and I was suffering with a heavy dose of the flu. I shouldn't have been at work but I turned up anyway because I love it. It was 11.30 a.m. and we were on air at noon. To prepare myself to get through the next six hours, I was lying on the floor of the broadcast box, trying to get a little sleep before the show began. Warren walked in, saw me on the floor and demanded to know why I was lying down. I told him I had the flu and was trying to get some sleep before we started on air. Wok didn't miss a beat: 'The flu, eh? Well get out of the box and down on the f**king sideline and have the flu down there.'

It was cold and wet and Warren had little interest in getting sick himself. I got a real insight into how he must have related to his players: the tough love. I can only imagine how brutal he was with anyone who bludged at training. I really hope Wok writes his own book one day. It would be a must-read for students of rugby league and students of life. I think I admire Wok so much because he has similar principles to my father.

Dad taught me to look people in the eye when I met them. Have a firm handshake, treat people how you would like to be treated and if you can't say something positive, shut up and say nothing. I'd recommend that to any young person, man or woman, trying to find a place in this world. The Wok is all about self-responsibility, self-discipline, harsh but fair criticism, large dollops of reality and a refusal to 'sugar-coat the bitter pill'. Perhaps without realising it, Wok has helped me through some very tough times. When I'm battling depression, he's one of the first people I trust to tell everything. When he asks how I'm going, if I'm feeling like crap, I tell him I'm feeling like crap. I know he appreciates the honesty.

I appreciate his willingness to hear the truth. He's played a big role in my learning the value of calling a spade a shovel. He has also been the person most responsible for educating me on the game of rugby league. In return, I think he's learned more about mental health, depression and bipolar disorder. He may not understand the issue completely (who does?) but Wok's willingness to try has meant a great deal. He's from a generation that used to dismiss it as hogwash.

Sports broadcaster David Morrow's help on the personal side has been immense. He'll get a phone call to say, look, Craig's not going too well at the moment, he has to give work a miss for a while. His sole concern is my welfare. Everything else is secondary. That's rare in the media—it can be a bloody ruthless business. People can turn on each other in a heartbeat. There'd be plenty of people in Dave's lofty position who, if their offsider pulled the pin on a game, would go through the roof. *How can Craig do this to me? How can he let me down again? I don't have a sideline eye, I don't have a co-host, I cannot work with this bloke any more.* Dave will call, wish me luck, say he'll see me again soon and he can't wait till we get the band back together. It's all I need to hear. I cannot tell Dave how much I appreciate it. Knowing someone cares when they don't have to gives you an enormous lift. That's mateship.

Dave is experienced enough to know the show will go on, which it always does—seamlessly. Like I say, no-one is irreplaceable, under any circumstances, least of all me. Dave's attitude is another reflection of the changing times. A sign there's a far greater understanding of mental illness. Dave is as old-school as Wok, a couple of no-nonsense individuals who may not have grown up with any real understanding of how debilitating a mental illness can be. It's not just the fact they've gained knowledge; it's that they've allowed their eyes and ears to be opened in the first place.

Will covering another Olympics make up for having missed out on the Sydney Games? Will that be my redemption? Not really. I'll never downplay how shattering it was in 2000. Even when I was in the psychiatric ward at James Fletcher Hospital and the Games had begun, even when I was extremely unwell with psychosis, I clung to this forlorn hope of checking out, getting back to Broadmeadow station, finally catch the XPT and making it to the Games, at least for the second week. Perhaps that was my most delusional thought of all. But when I watched Cathy Freeman win the 400 metres from my hospital bed, I knew it was all over. It was barely worth going anyway—the highlight of the whole Games, Cathy's win, had already come and gone. It took me a while to recover from the disappointment, frustration and anger, but it reaffirmed my belief that you can't win them all. If it's meant to happen, if I'm meant to get to an Olympics, I will, regardless of how much I scratch and claw for it. So I'm not going to scratch and claw at all.

I don't chase opportunities as hard as I used to. I'm available if I'm required. I'll always have my hand up but it's not all-consuming. I'm just as committed to working with mental health. Sports media is littered with reporters and commentators pushing each other over in the rush to cover a major event. I'm no longer one of them. My ego used to dictate that I chased the big-time opportunities. When I succeeded, I felt vindicated and puffed up. When I missed out, I felt robbed. I no longer want to feel puffed up. Those things are accomplishments and wonderful rewards, but they're not the be-all and end-all. The most important things in my life are my wife, my family, my friends and my health. Everything else is icing on the cake.

I'm proud to be on the ABC at all. I've covered sixteen straight rugby league grand finals. I have missed just one State of Origin since 1995. I'm blessed beyond all recognition. I love the ABC because we stand for something good. I'll keep turning up and doing my best. There's untold satisfaction in that. If missing the XPT in September 2000 means I've missed out on the Olympics forever, that's more than fine by me. I'll gladly just listen to Dave Morrow.

Feeling supported is more important, particularly if, just when things look to be sailing along very nicely, a storm cloud appears over the horizon.

The Black Dog comes back

As the years go by, more lows will come. Inevitably, inexorably, they will come, moving in like grim-faced soldiers in a black-and-white war movie. More highs will come, too, the smart alecs, traitors and liars. I'm ready for them both. Bring them on. I've grown accustomed to it. They have already reared their ugly heads at the most unexpected times . . .

It's late 2007 and 50 people are coming over for Christmas drinks. I've been looking forward to it for weeks, but shortly before everyone is due to arrive, I'm so depressed and flat, so stripped bare of energy and confidence, that I beg Louise to call the whole thing off. When the clouds move in like this, they're thick and suffocating and immoveable. Louise pays a price, too. Such a strain on everyone else, dull as dishwater. I'm so close to being the Grinch: I'm tempted to cancel Christmas, or a slice of it, in our house. The Christmas drinks are nearly cancelled, almost another casualty of this companion of mine, but in the end we carry on and I do my best to make out that things are fine.

It really is tough when you're in so low a mood. The most recent, unexpected blow-up was in early March 2010. I'm at lunch with a close circle of friends: Craig Eardley, Shivani Gupta and Melinda Smith. We always get together for a chat, 'The Meeting of the Minds', as we call it. We meet down near the Fishermen's Markets in Newcastle and chew the fat, tell each other what's happening in our own lives and solve the world's problems.

I'm taking it a little too literally on this day, escalating fast, climbing through lunch, talking way too much without listening to a single word being said by my friends. I'm preaching about spiritual matters with what I believe to be wise, deeply profound philosophical views. I want to do more than share them. I want to convince my rather shellshocked mates of them. I want to change their lives on the spot. They put up with me. Why, I do not know. Friendship in its purest form, I guess.

Lunch ends in a blur of my own overbearing rants. Melinda looks very concerned when it's time to leave. Craig is worried enough to ring my house later that afternoon to speak to Louise. He tells her how strangely I behaved at lunch and wants to know how I am. By four o'clock my pulse is racing, I'm having wild thoughts again. No religious imagery this time—I'm just plain paranoid: a surging feeling of dread. Something bad, horrifically and horrendously bad, is going to happen to me—I know it.

I'm trying to sit comfortably in the lounge room but my heart is going hammer and tongs. It's at that point, over a pot of tea that isn't having any sort of calming effect, when Louise puts down her cup and then her foot. Right, she says, we're going to James Fletcher. I agree to go. I trust her judgement completely . . . now.

It's called a waiting room for a reason. We sit there forever. The staff don't think it's an emergency because I don't have a broken bone, I'm not bleeding and there is no visible sign of injury. Mental health patients are put in the same waiting area as people with injured limbs, which makes no sense to me and ensures we're shoved to the back of the queue. Because I look OK, because I'm not screaming in agony or bleeding, they think I actually am OK. I'm not a priority even though Louise does her best to explain I'm spinning off my axis. I'm talking loudly and rapidly, there's a surprise.

Don't tell me it's not an emergency—it's a mental health emergency! It might not be life-threatening but leave it too long . . . I'm still armed with an unshakable opinion on every topic under the sun. I understand the world, the cosmos and the universe better than anyone else and I must ram it down everyone else's naive throats. Louise keeps checking my pulse. More questions. 'What are you thinking?'

'Nothing.'

'Come on, what are you thinking?'

'Everything.'

'Why do I have to explain it? Don't you see what's going on here? Isn't it obvious? I'm on an extremely important spiritual mission.' But then paranoia returns. I can't get better. I just can't get better. Help me.

I'm lucid enough to know my thoughts are out of whack. Now I'm agitated and irrational and delusional. We wait and wait and wait.

It's absurd: welcome to the public health system.

Louise ends up begging for someone to see me before I land in another full-blown psychosis. Finally a member of staff in the emergency department realises that we actually do have an emergency with this soon-to-be totally psychotic man. 'What are you thinking, Craig? Tell me!' Finally, I own up.

This is fairly disconcerting. I tell Louise that if I am admitted to this hospital, if I have to spend so much as one night in a ward, I will be murdered. The staff will kill me in my sleep. Once again I am experiencing a psychotic episode, which is a detachment from reality. It's not much fun, to say the least.

While I can look back on these experiences with a good deal of dispassion now, it does take some time. I've found that one of the great things about life is that just around the corner is another opportunity. Find an inner peace and you don't have to travel too far to experience it.

28 Nine and a half kilometres

Only since my diagnosis have I started looking after myself. Only now do I look after myself properly. My first internal check-up comes as soon as I open my eyes in the morning. Where am I today? How am I really travelling? High road? Low road? How am I *really* feeling? It has to be real: honesty with myself is paramount otherwise the whole process is waste of time. A ludicrous part of pride is that sometimes not only do we steer clear of admitting our distresses to the people whose approval we seek, but we're just as reluctant to come clean to ourselves. I run through my checklist of questions and answer them honestly. I think a lot of these routines are beneficial to everyone, not just people with mental illnesses. We all need to keep an eye on ourselves. If I'm not running around like a lunatic, or if I'm not dragging my heels and struggling to find the motivation to simply get out of bed and face the day, I know I'm ready to roll.

Diet-wise, I'm imperfect, but I do try. I eat fewer processed foods than before. Raw natural oatmeal is sprinkled on my cereal every morning. I've slashed my coffee intake. When I first started in the media, I regularly drank five cups a day, two sugars in each. It was enough to blow my head off: a state of being, back then, I found appealing. That was too much caffeine and sugar,

too much fake energy. The slump would come in the late afternoon, further proof that highs always lead to lows, ups necessitate
downs; the whole lot a balancing act, a nonstop game of give and
take, 24 hours a day, seven days a week.

I'm down to one coffee a day, occasionally two. I enjoy it
because I just love a good coffee. I savour the smell and the
taste and the gentle kick because I'm not slamming them down
nonstop. It's got to be espresso and it has to be of the highest
quality. I'm not interested in the instant stuff. I gave that up a
long time ago.

> 'All men should strive to learn before they die what
> they are running from, and to, and why.'
> James Thurber

I have no sugar and feel a million bucks for it. I felt terrible
without it for the first few weeks and definitely had withdrawal
symptoms but I persevered . . . now I don't even think about
having sugar. It's helped to even out my mood, as I'm no longer
veering between an energy hit from the sugar followed by a
slump when the effect wears off. I started cutting back by only
having half a sugar.

The people at my local cafe, 3 Bean, start making my espresso
as soon as I walk through the door. I like that. If I were somewhere else, in Sydney for instance, I'd get these strange looks in
the cafes down there: you want *half* a sugar? You want me to open
this sachet and pour in only *half*? Yes, thanks champ. That's exactly
what I want you to do. They roll their eyes. I couldn't care less.
Ask for half a sugar, you get half a sugar. Now there's none at all.
Quitting caffeine altogether is probably the ideal but I'm not as
determined in that regard as Mark Gable. I'll never give up my
daily hit. I'm a man with bipolar, not a Buddhist monk.

When it comes to fitness, my routine varies. The problem is

that I get very bored, very easily. Swimming laps bores me stupid. I chop and change my routines to keep them fresh. Being at the beach, kicking off my shoes and going barefoot: that raw, earthy feeling of sand beneath my feet and between my toes is tremendously grounding when I'm feeling disconnected.

I chop and change my routines to keep them fresh.

Everyone needs a special routine and place; one thing they know will make them feel completely free of worry. Mine is a 9.5 kilometre stretch of bliss, a meditation session with exercise—the best of both worlds. Even better: a meditation session without actually going into a meditative state. Louise's brother, Matthew, introduced me to the 90-minute walk from Newcastle's Ocean Baths to Merewether Beach and back. This is my sanctuary most Saturday mornings, so therapeutic that I spend the rest of the week looking forward to going back there.

From the baths, I walk up over Strzelecki Hill and down in front of the picture-perfect stretch of coastline that is Bar Beach, The Cliff, Dixon Park and Merewether, four beaches lined up in front of me like a string of diamonds. Strzelecki is a pretty steep climb. The view from the other side is breathtaking and the reward for having conquered it. On a sunny day, the water a luminescent blue, there's no place on earth I would rather be. I stop at the bubbler, get a drink—even the drink thrills me because it's all part of the routine.

I can taste how good the water is before I open my mouth. I can taste it on a Tuesday when my mind wanders back. I keep moving with a brain that tends to think about a whole lot of things at once, veering off in different directions without any instructions to do so. It's not necessarily a bad thing to have all these ideas zapping around in my head but it needs to be put on pause for a while.

The Bathers Way does it for me. Before then, dizzying is the right word to describe the stuff pinging round in there, an indecipherable blur of ideas. Focusing on one can be like looking out the window of a speeding car and trying to photograph a tree. There's nothing wrong with having big ideas and a creative mind but it needs to be controlled and organised. Those of us with bipolar, we're in good company. 'Madness comes from God, whereas sober sense is merely human,' Socrates said in his speech on divine madness in Plato's *Phaedrus*. Another quote, from Aristotle, comes to mind: 'Why is it that all men who are outstanding in philosophy, poetry and the arts are melancholic?'

On today's walk I'm fascinated by the list of famous figures either known to have been bipolar, or were thought to have ridden the wave: poets self-medicating their depression with opium and alcohol; artists such as Vincent Van Gogh and Edvard Munch using their swinging moods to fire their creative drive. The tempestuousness. The list of musicians is endless: Kurt Cobain, who took his own life; Nina Simone, Axl Rose and Sinéad O'Connor.

In truth, we don't know the half of it: bipolar hadn't been defined when some of history's most confounding creatives were alive. Retrospective diagnoses have come thick and fast based on the timelines of their bodies of work and anecdotal evidence of their behaviour. What they did but, most importantly, when they did it.

For these people, manic periods of almost superhuman productivity were followed by periods of bleak nothingness. Oscar Wilde: if he wasn't bipolar, I don't know who is. Some of his more eccentric behaviours were known at the time, but they weren't written about as mania or bipolar. Take the composer, Mahler. He wrote 50 concertos in seven months. Impossible. He went from being frenetic and unstoppable to having six months in which he did nothing at all. Abraham Lincoln was desperately depressed. Winston Churchill, of course, summed up depression like no-one else ever has, so succinctly and perfectly: 'It is the Black Dog.' Churchill ended up having to take a bottle of whisky to bed with him. That was his method of coping. If a man as brilliant as Winston Churchill needed to be sedated in that way, and to do it himself, there's no greater illustration of the helplessness it can conjure.

None of these brilliant people would have admitted to psychosis because there would have been no understanding of it. Take today's stigma and multiply it by a million. The relationship between mental illness and extravagant works seems real to me. Not because I can create anything remotely comparable, but because if I was trained in the arts or music, I can *imagine,* when escalating, having the energy to pump out endless works. We can never really know, but I'm guessing such other-worldly productivity needs some out-of-the-ordinary psychological phases.

There are too many links for it to be a coincidence, too many 'smoking guns'. Take Beethoven's large-scale works of heroism and struggle; periods of low and high productivity. Tolstoy, the Russian novelist, was suicidal when he couldn't reconcile his faith with the material world. 'Everybody thinks of changing humanity and nobody thinks of changing himself,' he wrote. He was grappling with forces outside his control. I wonder how they would have fared in the modern day.

The sensory overload of bipolar can be overwhelming but I know when I need to pull back, take my time, marvel at the natural beauty in the world. When I'm walking along The Bathers Way, I just have to look left and there it is—calm. The overload is swallowed by the sea. What an incredible effect. What fantastic perspective the ocean provides. It reminds me of the endless parts of the world, all the way out to the horizon and beyond, that don't revolve around me. Every day is different: the varying sizes of the waves; there might be 30 ships on the horizon or there might be none; the beach might be packed with people or it might be empty. It might be a sunbaked 30-degree day, it could be a bitter nine degrees, but the routine never changes—that's the important thing.

These 9.5 kilometres are freedom and clarity and the kill switch inside my brain when there's too much going on. I can't stop it myself, and that's been important to realise. I need help and happily seek it. It's neither a weakness nor an admission of defeat. It's empowering to find assistance in your own little ways. The Bathers Way: at times when I need proof the sun really does come up every morning, I look left and there it is.

Halfway along the walk, at the bottom of the Merewether steps, silver foxes are standing in their Speedos, getting their morning sun. They're so relaxed, talking with slow, lazy smiles, leaning back against the warm concrete wall to be soaked in sunshine. Whether they realise it or not, they're meditating. The simple things are so good, so perfect! Half the joy is in realising exactly how simple it can all be. Anyone can find their own slice of nirvana. Away from the coast, mountains have the same effect as the sea, or rivers, or lakes, or landscapes or the tranquillity of isolated areas: a desert can be the most soulful place of all.

Looking at the rolling waves, getting some sun, powering through wind and rain so strong I can barely see, just casting everything aside for a while—nothing beats it for me. There's a blackboard at Merewether with the day's water temperature on it. Thanks to whoever writes it up there every morning. It's another tidbit that excites me: something else I can rely on, another mark in the road—and it lets me know, especially on the bitterly cold winter mornings, what I'm in for when I take the plunge back at the Newcastle baths. In summer the water temperature will be between 18 and 21 degrees Celsius; in winter it might get down to 14 or 15.

Life is a matter of working out what brings you the most

joy and doing it as often as possible. Is it not that simple? Do we not complicate it too much? These sources of the sublime aren't the big extravagances, the near-impossible things to attain. The Bathers Way does not cost me one cent, yet the value to my peace of mind is immeasurable. Do the things you enjoy. Turn your back on the stuff you don't. Piece of cake. It's only taken me 49 years to work that out!

Merewether's blackboard is halfway along The Bathers Way. I turn past the silver foxes in their Speedos and head back towards Strzelecki. Everything at Bar Beach can have changed by the time I return. The wind might have picked up or dropped off, the tide might have shifted a bit, clouds might have gathered or disappeared—it's a reminder of the impermanence of all that we see, think and feel. Everything shall pass. I get so invigorated. So refreshed and inspired.

Never will I walk The Bathers Way with an iPod blaring in my ears. My phone is off or absent. I don't want to be taking calls, I don't want any artificial noise, I just want to find my peace. People stride along wearing headphones and I can hear the heavy metal, it's that loud. Don't get me wrong. I love music. It's the scripture of life. Midnight Oil, Johnny Cash, Fleetwood Mac, Cold Chisel, Jackson Browne: I love them. But not now. I don't want any of them on the Bathers Way with me. They'll defeat the purpose, deny me the full natural experience. I'm doing a weekly spring clean, getting rid of the clutter. It's brilliant: I'm making more room for the stuff I need and want. I see a lot of people on The Bathers Way getting the exercise part, and that's great, but they're clogging their brains rather than clearing them out. It's as if those headphone wearers are scared of their own thoughts and need the heavy metal to take their mind off the fact that they're alone with their deepest thoughts. They're not enjoying the view, they're not getting the chance to enjoy the sights and sounds around them, the waves running up the shore.

I find calm in the steadiness of my own footsteps. I have started to like time spent with myself. It's a great challenge to keep your own company. It can be frightening but it has to be learned. Without an iPod, or music or phone calls, I'm getting the full experience.

I've started plenty of these walks in a restless mood but I've never finished in anything other than great spirits. I'm so into it I forget that I'm actually getting exercise in the process. The heart rate is up without it being too much of a hard slog. How good is this? That's what I'm thinking, and what I want to be thinking as often as possible till the time comes to draw my last breath: how good is this! Back up Strzelecki, another stop at the beloved bubbler, back down the steps, back past King Edward Park, back to the Newcastle Ocean Baths. I've got a good core body temperature worked up by now, even in winter.

I grab my swimmers out of the car, get changed as fast as I can and dive straight in, regardless of whether the water is icy or idyllic. I think diving into the water is a metaphor. I know I want to do something, but if I think about it too much, if I dwell on it for too long, I'll find reasons not to and it won't happen. The water's too cold. I don't want to get a headache. I'll catch the flu. I just don't need this. I'd better play it safe and stay up here where it's warm and risk-free. I've found that when I throw myself into the deep end—in the Newcastle Ocean Baths and in life—more often than not, I'm glad that I did.

The cold water jolts me. I've never felt so alive. I walk up and down the pool a few times, a bit of a recovery session for the legs. I'm in one big ice bath. I stay in for ten minutes or so, the cold making my skin crackle and pop with energy. I understand now why surfers become so addicted to the rush of their dawn patrols. The first wash of salt water across my face is extraordinarily cleansing. In winter I climb out of the pool with the wind chill whistling and the temperature skidding to about seven degrees. That's a *maximum* of seven. Straight under a hot shower in the change rooms. (Plenty of ocean baths and beaches don't have hot showers, but Newcastle does.)

It's a great challenge to keep your own company.

There's no feeling to compare with warm water on cold skin. The raw, edgy vitality it provides. I can feel it from head to toe, endorphins releasing this incredible charge of energy, and it's natural. It's not plus-four, that bastard, it's not the effect of alcohol, it's a purely natural high. There's no pain, no turmoil. I feel brand new, completely re-energised.

Getting into the car to drive off, I'm already thinking that I can't wait for next Saturday. The buzz lasts an entire day. I have a coffee and it tastes like the best damn coffee I've ever had in my life. A deep breath and the realisation that *everything* is great. I'm relaxed, alive, alert, every cobweb blown (and washed) away. Thoughts are clear and concise. I will continue to do this walk whenever possible and find some new ones to experience as well. And I'll continue to look for other ways to support my health and wellbeing.

29 The miracle of yoga

There's many reasons yoga works. I'm concentrating so hard on the different asanas, the different positions, both getting into them then trying desperately to untangle myself back out, that I completely forget about all the other junk clunking around in my head. I've gone to a yoga class with a million things on my mind—and walked out singing.

A 90-minute yoga session makes a significant difference to my mental, physical and spiritual wellbeing. Don't be scared by the thought that you might be hopeless at it. That you're so unfit and out-of-shape you'll embarrass yourself. I was hopeless when I first started and I'm still no Indian Rubber Man, but I get as much benefit as anyone.

Your level of expertise, even if that level is zero, makes no difference. Ten years ago I was the worst in the class and probably still am. Make yourself go once a week for six weeks and the results will blow your mind. Yoga can twist and turn itself to fit most budgets. Classes are easy to find: newspaper advertisements, internet searches, community noticeboards.

If you look for a yoga class, you'll find one. Mine is at a senior citizens centre in Newcastle. We get about 40 people in the hall on a timber floor. I take my mat, and a towel, pay my sixteen bucks, follow the instructor's advice and I'm away. Nothing makes me feel better than this. I just listen and fall into my own little trance.

Another silver lining is that it helps keep me physically fit. Other therapies are my back-ups to yoga. I bring them into play when I'm not feeling so well. Yoga is the constant. I'm committed to it for the rest of my life. Foolishly, I gave it up for three years a while back for the same reason we cease doing a lot of things that are good for us. We get too busy. I got too smart for my own good, thinking I knew everything about bipolar when really, I didn't. I prioritised poorly. My work–life balance went down the chute.

Some lessons needed to be re-learned. When this happens, they are forged in steel. I had become complacent, thinking I had better things to do than get in the car and drive across town to a yoga class. I skipped one session, let another slip and suddenly I had gone three years without doing a yoga class. I thought I didn't need it any more. I thought my bipolar was under control.

When the clouds started to strangle me again, when I was so far down the low road I was starting to think I might never get back up, I knew what I had to do. Getting back to my yoga classes was among my highest priorities. As we were signing in, a woman in my class said, 'Are you Craig Hamilton?' She said she'd got into yoga because she had read my story about how crucial yoga had become in my life. She was in her 30s, maybe early 40s, and had never properly committed to it previously. After reading my first book, she adopted the six-week test and has been going ever since, unable to imagine life without it. She attends more than I do.

I challenge you to find anyone whose life has been wrecked by yoga. While you're relaxing in the yoga class, be conscious of staying in the present moment.

30 Learning to chill

When I want to really relax, I sit or lie down, close my eyes, and listen to a guided meditation. Nothing is rushed. My breathing is slow and deep. In through the nose and out through the mouth. It can take as few as three breaths for complete relaxation to wash over me. I think we forget about the very powerful effect breathing has on our body and state of mind.

In a guided meditation, you close your eyes and focus on the voice of your guide. *You're relaxing your fingers . . . relaxing your hands . . .* You'll be talked through each body part: fingers, backs of the hands, fronts of the hands, elbows, shoulders, neck, right through to your toes. It can be done either with a practitioner face to face or by following prompts on a recording.

In guided meditation I never quite fall asleep, but come very close in such a dreamy state. Most yoga classes provide guided meditation for the same cost as a yoga session. At around sixteen dollars, that's dirt cheap for the rewards. When I do it, all I can hear, all I can think about, is the voice of the guide and the absolute relaxation flowing through my body. The first time I ever experienced a guided meditation session was with another gifted therapist, Glenda Schmidt, who is based in Newcastle.

The calm experienced afterwards was amazing. The effects can be long-lasting, but regular practice is the key . . . once a week is ideal.

31 Emotional freedom technique (EFT)

As you've probably already gathered, an extension of my spiritual exploration and search for wellbeing has been the discovery of alternative therapies. My mates will be rolling round laughing when they read about this because I used to swear till I was luminescent blue in the face that such far-out treatments were only for hippies and freaks; that they're performed by modern-day witch doctors. You want to stick a needle in my head and another in my big toe? Pass.

However, I've gone from scepticism to being a true believer. I'm really conscious of not shoving these ideas down your throat because not everyone does cartwheels when I tell them about yet another therapy that has given me goosebumps, but give them a go. You might hate them. You might think they are the most ridiculous things you have ever done in your life. You might even think I'm delusional right now for even suggesting them—but one or two might just have your name on them.

Personally, I cannot recommend these therapies highly enough. I wouldn't waste your time by suggesting them if I didn't have proof they work. No-one was more reluctant than I before I tried them. During my first session of reiki, for instance, I was on the verge of bursting out laughing and bolting for the door. But here

I am, imploring you to give a few of the therapies I talk about in this book a try, mental illness or not.

My plan was to list the pros and cons of each—but I couldn't think of any cons. I will say that finding the right practitioner is important: someone you're comfortable explaining your situation to. The more the specialist knows, the more he or she can help.

One such treasured discovery for me is Emotional Freedom Technique (EFT). Not heard of it? Jump on YouTube, type it in and a qualified practitioner will give you an introduction. You'll be an expert in an hour. EFT targets energy blockages that stem from anxiety. We don't understand how these anxieties grow, or where they've come from, but we know they're unpleasant and need to be shifted. It's a very powerful tool that can be largely self-administered once you know what to do. I perform it on myself with occasional visits to a specialist. Being able to self-administer EFT at 2 a.m., 2 p.m. or right this very second is fantastic. However, it is expensive, so if it's going to wipe out other treatments, EFT can't be your psychological weapon of choice.

The technique involves tapping the meridian points on your body with your index and middle finger while repeating a mantra. (A friend or family member can do the honours if you don't want to do it yourself.) You can make up your own mantra, or steal mine: *Even though I'm feeling anxious and depressed, I love and accept myself.*

It sounds absurd—but then it starts to sink in. I start to like it. Who cares if it sounds dicky? It's important. For me, the first meridian point is the spot above my right eyebrow. Next is the right cheekbone, basically the bottom of my eye socket. Then above my top lip. Beneath my bottom lip, more or less tapping the top of my chin. The collarbone. The final spot to be tapped is the rib cage, beneath my arm.

If I don't feel any difference the first time I do it, I try again. The less experienced you are, the more repetitions it might take. Initially it took me three or four goes to stop feeling like the village idiot, but it does work. I really did think it was the stupidest thing I had ever done (well, since reiki) when I first went to see a specialist practitioner I found on the internet. She started tapping me on the head like she was thinking, *Hello, anyone in there?*

I was obediently saying my mantra like a school kid being forced to repeat his times tables. The words were coming out of my mouth, but inside I was cringing. I was embarrassed to think my life had come to this. I thought, seriously, if only my old mates could see me now. I couldn't connect with it, nearly biting my fist to stop myself laughing but after our fourth routine, lo and behold, I started to feel incredibly calm.

At this stage I had fairly acute feelings of depression. I was so down and lacking in confidence. What EFT achieved after three or four repeats, one straight after the other, was incredible. Each time, the practitioner would say: 'On a scale of one to ten, how would you rate your emotions now?' (Ten being the most intensely bad feelings; one being the calm you're chasing.) Each time, the number I told her had reduced. I was eight out of ten when we started, really strung out. Then it was six, five, three, my mood levelling to a very noticeable degree. I was stunned. Midway through the session, I felt like laughing for a different reason: this works!

I was introduced to EFT by an amazing lady named Joanne Antoun. Joanne is an incredibly multifaceted therapist who I still see occasionally when I need a tune-up. It takes time to get used to. Something about saying you love yourself makes us all cringe. My answer to that is this: somebody has to.

32 No, not the needles!

The most unexpected avenues can be life-changing. Initially my attitude was: 'No, not the needles!' Acupuncture wasn't for me. I assumed it would be painful. (That was wrong assumption #3457.) Having always hated needles, the thought of paying a stranger to stick them into me held little appeal, but so many people recommended it that I decided to give it a go. And what I've discovered is it's highly effective in healing physical injuries and soothing the mind—and it doesn't hurt a bit. Like EFT, it's a great way to find balance by unblocking meridians. I now try to go once a month.

On my first visit, I explained to the therapist that I had bipolar disorder and wanted to work on my energy balance. When I told him that, he instantly said: 'Right, I know how I can treat you.'

Very fine needles went into the underneath of my knee, a couple in my stomach—just tiny pinpricks. Simply by checking my pulse, the therapist could tell exactly where they had to go. 'Righto,' he said, 'you've got a bit of congestion around the kidney and your liver; you've got problems with your digestive tract.' He'd place a needle in my leg, thigh, stomach or between my shoulder blades.

I'm glad I told the therapist my whole story. Tell your own specialist as much as you can. It can only help. Sometimes when I go in, he checks my pulse and it's really flat. I might be acting upbeat but as soon as he takes my pulse, he knows I'm running low. He knows I'm faking.

If I'm riding high, my pulse racing, he knows how to bring me down. He treats both ends of the spectrum, both polarities, through different meridian points. He's stuck a needle into a toe to the point where it's drawn blood. He's stuck a needle in my big toe while placing another in the top of my head, right at the crown. You might think that's impossible, that our heads are too hard, but the needles are superfine.

Acupuncture has been really helpful in keeping me on an even keel. It's become a terrific maintenance treatment to ensure that whether I'm down or up, the scales return to balance. And when I'm feeling well, it's ensured I keep feeling well, although I have to be careful about distractions because as soon as I walk out the door, they'll be there. They can creep up on us easily. Quite often that distraction might be the phone we carry around in our pockets.

33 (Anti)social media

If you want to be more relaxed then it's important to work out where your stressors are and do something about them. I might be a dinosaur but I have a beef with technology: I reckon it's a big stress factor for many of us. I know Facebook and Twitter are part of the e-revolution and that there are pluses, such as increased convenience and immediacy, but for all the upsides, there are also alarming downsides with consequences for mental health. Social media is supposed to make us more connected, but I believe it's responsible for a sense of disconnection, thanks to the anxieties it creates. I doubt 'social media' is the right term, either, because what we're being suckered into doesn't seem all that social to me.

These sites, and the devices that make access to them so super-easy, are threatening to dominate our lives to the extent that they *become* our lives. I know people who spend more time on Facebook than they do on anything else. That's no way to live. It's not living at all, the claustrophobic opposite to my nine-and-a-half kilometres of freedom. Generation Y in particular has to find a way to extricate itself from electronics before their lives become insular and narrow-minded.

'To err is human, but to really foul things up requires a computer.'

Paul R. Ehrlich

The world is a large and wondrous place. We have uniquely brilliant and fascinating people all around us. Every single one of us is different, we all have incredible stories but we spend more time steering clear of each other than getting to know one another. All I see is people with their heads buried in smartphones and iPads. Check out the public transport system. Everyone is looking down instead of up. It's not just teenagers I'm talking about here. An adult couple is sitting on a park bench: they should be talking or cuddling but all they're doing is scrolling through their iPhones. That frustrates me.

One day we'll look back on the wasted moments and wish we'd made more of them. One thing I have learned is that our very existence is a gift—a miracle—but some are missing it. They're texting instead of talking. They have a thousand Facebook 'friends' but nobody they can really talk to. Instead of delivering real praise to someone, they hit 'Like' and move on.

I agree that social media and technology have their place in our lives—I use them myself—but we have to start controlling them instead of letting them rule over us. There needs to be balance. This isn't a tirade against all forms of social media. In my view, the issue is overuse.

To me they lack *substance*, covering the cracks and relieving boredom. They're great in moderation but they're not terribly enriching to the spirit. I'm still working out how to manoeuvre them to my own advantage. I want *them* to help *me*.

I don't like the diminished levels of human contact. I'm convinced our agitation levels have increased as a result. Our souls are crying out for the human touch but we're getting further away. It impacts on physical health and emotional functioning. I can be as guilty as anyone as falling into the trap but I have realised, in more recent times, the importance of rebelling against it.

I like tuning in to get a quick glimpse, find what I have to and get off before I get burned. The distractions and temptations are endless. Twenty minutes on Facebook can become two hours and there goes the neighbourhood. Two hours can become six hours and an entire day is wasted. Then a week. You wake up exhausted because somehow you were still on the net at 1 a.m. When I go to bed at night, I don't want to be thinking about how I've spent most of my day on Twitter and Facebook. Ditto for when I'm on my deathbed. What did I do with my life? Well, spent a lot of time on the computer . . . no thanks.

Anyone *really* having the time of their life, anyone really on top of the world and secure enough in themself to be content with the present moment, isn't sending out a barrage of Twitter messages or Facebook updates. Are we trying to convince everyone that our shortcomings don't exist? In researching for this book I've read a lot of Facebook posts, and tweets, that leave me with the impression that the author is trying desperately to impress everyone. That they're sweating on people hitting the 'Like' or 'Retweet' button as a form of validation. It sounds to me like they're trying to convince themselves more than anyone else.

All the thoughts and emotions and abilities already inside us, aren't they enough? It's a massive problem: we're losing the ability to entertain ourselves. We're used to having ten different conversations going at once, TV on in the background, music in the other background, Facebook and Twitter and YouTube all running at the same time on split screens—and we wonder why we can't get to sleep at night. Our brains are frying—I don't think they know how to handle it all.

Multi-tasking might be a skill, but surely that skill can be used in better ways than this. I'm not going to bank on electronic devices for my happiness. Gen Y wants fast and furious action, all day every day, coming at them from every angle. They demand to be entertained—and then they're barely able to say a single word in conversation. Their internet identities have become their real identities. That's got trouble, in the form of depression later in their lives, written all over it.

We're designed to connect to people instead of appliances. Nothing breaks my heart more than hearing about teenagers holed up at home on a computer or phone when the sun's shining outside. Adults should know better than to let them. Problem being, we're doing it ourselves. We're getting told every day that Australians are becoming more obese. This is leading to increased blood-pressure levels, diabetes issues, heart disease. And we ask ourselves, why? Poor diet is a big part of it, but the lack of exercise is integral, and what causes that? Electronics. Playing computer tennis instead of the real thing. I really don't want to sound like a dinosaur here but back in my day, we'd run around from daylight to dusk.

Being fit was normal and the by-product of our physical habits—how we lived our lives, how we grew up—lasted a life-time. Before school, after school, weekend and holidays, we were going nonstop. We were active. Why? Because it was fun. We were spending time with people whose company we enjoyed, our mates. We fed off each other's enthusiasm. We were using our imaginations to invent new games, finding ways to keep ourselves amused. Hide-and-seek would never have been invented in the computer age. No game nowadays is as fun as that.

These days a kid can spend dawn-to-dusk playing computer games. No sunlight. He or she turns the computer off, has a fat-filled dinner and goes to bed. The mind and body are screaming *no!* Australia used to be filled with kids playing backyard cricket and footy. Plenty are still involved in organised sport, training a couple of days a week and playing on the weekends. I think those people stand out like sore thumbs. They look fresh, vital and healthy.

The lazier, stay-indoors me isn't half the person that the sport-playing, exercising me is. I've started playing cricket on the weekends again and I'm all the better for it. Between the slothful Craig and the energetic Craig, I know which version is better.

34 Confessions of the preacher

As well as having Facebook and Twitter accounts, I have a mobile phone sitting in my pocket right now. If it beeps, rings, buzzes or does whatever it does, I will probably answer it. But I don't have a smartphone—by choice. People see my ancient mobile, look at me mournfully, shake their heads in commiseration. Poor bloke, your phone's about ten years old! Bet it doesn't even have an app! I really don't want emails and the internet on my phone. It's a telephone. I want to make and receive telephone calls. Text messaging is the extent of the extras I want. Because that's all I need to communicate.

Everything else is a waste of time, and I don't have enough left in this lifetime to waste. Emails can wait till I'm sitting in front of a computer at work—or at home when I need to. I'm protecting myself against myself: because I can see myself, very easily, falling into the very patterns I've been criticising.

That's been a joy in getting to know myself a bit better. I know the safety measures I need. I don't want to become a victim of technology. I try to limit my time on Facebook to twenty minutes per day. Sometimes I'll go over that, but only just. Sometimes I won't get on at all and that night I'll be feeling very good about it, almost proud. You didn't get me today! I'm exercising control over my life.

I give myself ten or fifteen minutes a day on Twitter. I don't trawl through all the tweets, as that would take too long. It comes in handy as a way to network; I can put material on there relating to the ABC's broadcasts, put out information on a public talk I might be giving. I try to put a few inspirational quotes out there, too.

There are some great sites to follow on Twitter: iamsource, Greatest Quotes. They're examples of Twitter being used to inspire. I like reading these motivational quotes first thing in the morning, they rev me up. You can get the wisdom of every-one from Socrates and Plato to Abraham Lincoln and Winston Churchill. No harm done there. They make me *think*. Most of all, they make me want to think about actually living what I've just read.

Imagine this scene. I'm sure you'll recognise this. You're out at a restaurant in the company of two, four, six friends, having a lovely meal, enjoying the group you're with. There'll be a group on another table. Someone's phone will go off and it'll be an email or a call—and the whole conversation and vibe comes to a crash-ing halt. The person is immersed in their iPhone while they're supposed to be enjoying the company of friends. They've virtu-ally walked out on everyone at their table and entered cyberspace. Come on. How rude and disrespectful is that? They're saying hang on, something more important than this conversation, someone more important than you, needs me. I'll only give you my atten-tion when there's no-one else who wants to get in touch.

Seriously, it's so bloody rude and antisocial. Who's so impor-tant that you have to offend friends by not giving them your full attention? If the person in your phone is so special, go and have dinner with them! How wonderful it would be if we all turned off our phones every time we sat down to meet.

I'm very conscious of how much time is being spent on these distractions. Instead, I want more of what will enrich me. How much of your life, day by day, is social media chewing up? For me, it used to be too much. I'd never have read *Autobiography of a Yogi* if I'd been on Facebook. I want to re-engage with my family, re-engage with the world around me. Imagine watching all this from another planet, trying to work out how human beings behave. Imagine watching more than a billion of us hunched over our little machines in self-absorbed silence. *That* is madness.

The Lakeside Hilton

MARCH 2010. The more I understand the journey, the more I can go with it, rather than battle it. Finally, I'm assessed. Finally I'm medicated and admitted to the Calvary Mater Hospital, the newly opened public mental health hospital in Newcastle. The system has to do better than this. People with mental illness, and their families, should be spared even one second of delay. I wake the next morning with air in my lungs. The nurses have decided against murdering me. I think this is a positive way to start the day. I'm then moved to the Lakeside Private Psychiatric Hospital at Warners Bay.

If you want a model of what a first-class modern psychiatric hospital should be, check in and check it out. Others are too confronting, dire, backward, harsh, stuck in the 1950s. Lakeside is state of the art. For starters, it's bright. It has flowers. Some mental health hospitals don't have a single flower, and they are drab and dull. What, people with mental illness don't deserve some flowers in our rooms?

Lakeside feels like a plush hotel . . . relaxing, exactly what we need. We get the feeling of being looked after by people who actually care, staff with an interest in what we're going through, treating us as human beings instead of whatever label we may have attained from our condition. The accommodation at Lakeside, the quality of staff, the facility itself, the care, the professionalism in terms of the bread and butter of getting the medications exactly right, I cannot speak highly enough of Lakeside. Comfortable common areas have lounge chairs and big-screen TVs. It gets pretty interesting, though, because there are two very separate groups of patients with two very different sets of mental states. Lakeside gives an opportunity to the manic, and the depressed, to choose their common rooms.

There's the low room and the high room. I've only been in the latter. What a hoot! I've never been hospitalised when depressed, only when higher than a Goodyear blimp. With depression, I just endure. I get home care. I take my medication, stay in touch with my doctor, do all my therapies, swim in the icy water, dive into yoga, keep my head down, try to keep my chin up, and remember that this too will pass. I look for joy anywhere I can find it—a patch of blue sky, a cool breeze. I ride out the storm.

Every hour conquered is a win. Rack up enough wins and I'm clear. I don't know about the low room at Lakeside, but across the corridor: man, the up room is buzzing! We're flying, waiting to be medicated down but it's taking a while. We're watching TV, laughing and joking, having a whale of a time. No damage can be done because we're in a controlled environment. I can only imagine what the scene would look like to an outside observer: New Year's Eve right on midnight, but the stroke of midnight lasts all day.

In the other room are the depressed. The manic room is too noisy and hyper for them so they get their own area. Not such a hoot in there, obviously—rather funereal, really, but vitally important. Misery doesn't mind a bit of company, as they say. Lakeside deserves credit for acknowledging the different needs of the two extremes. In the public system, everyone is thrown into the one area. If you're down or you're up, too bad. It can feel wrong and inappropriate. You feel guilty, in a bizarre way, that you're high while others are so low. The depressed feel awkward and self-conscious, retreating to their own rooms and staying there. Sometimes you just need to be alone in that condition.

Lakeside has computers, internet connection and the food is outstand-ing compared to public hospital food which, to put it in the most glowing terms, is adequate. Lakeside's catering is top-shelf. So irresistible that I put on weight while I'm in there. The medication I'm on doesn't help in the weight department. Zyprexa is notorious for increasing appetite. They've got juice 24/7. Tea and coffee. You walk past the bar and make yourself a cup of whatever you want. Everyone sits together for meals, which I think is great therapy in itself, a bit of camaraderie.

For every one of my hospitalisations, another twenty to 25 people have been with me. I've met some fascinating people with incredible life stories behind the walls of psychiatric hospitals. The clientele is diverse: high achievers, non-achievers, people from all walks of life and profes-sions. A guy from the armed forces. A police officer. Uni students, school kids, a teenager in Year 12 getting ready for her HSC. We receive fabulous care. I'm discharged and go home. I've become comfortable with bipolar being a cyclical illness. This isn't the beginning or end of anything. It's just another phase.

There are periods when I'm fighting fit, mentally and physically, for months and even years on end. But I have come to learn that nothing, good or bad, lasts forever. I've been privileged enough to speak at Lakeside for the opening of a new wing. I stood there and said, 'You know, the last time I was here, I was a patient.' People laughed—until they realised I was serious.

35 Finding your way out

When we're in a bad space it's easy to assume there's no help available, yet we don't hesitate to get help for a broken arm or leg, for a problem with our eyesight or hearing. Mental illness is just another part of us that goes wrong. It's made a big difference to me since I've realised this, and also realised that I can't get through it on my own. How those around us react once they understand we're struggling with mental issues can have a huge impact on whether we get proper help, whether we stay on our medication, whether we take good care of ourselves. This brave letter I received some time back helps put all this in perspective.

I am elderly now. I had a brother who suffered from manic depression. He died at the age of 80 and has been dead for a number of years. He became manic depressive at the age of 50 and for a decade or so was a big problem for his wife and family until he was put on lithium, which was very successful in controlling his mood swings. For the last years of his life he was able to live almost normally. He lived in the country so I'm not sure that he had the most up-to-date medical treatment.

However, what I am really writing about is your view that mental illness should not be treated differently from physical illness as far as it is open to the public and not considered a taboo topic which has to be hidden away. When I was five my mother became epileptic and

I still have a sister who suffered epilepsy from her early twenties. I have always held very strongly to the view that the only way to get rid of the taboo placed on sufferers of mental illness is to talk openly about these illnesses in the same way that people speak openly of illness in general.

So where's the way forward? I hope and believe mental illness will be bracketed with physical illnesses one day. Not many agree with me, but I hope it's just a matter of when. The bubonic plague killed millions of people. So did smallpox. Cholera still kills in third-world countries. Bipolar disorder? There will be a cure for it like there's a cure for other physical illnesses. I will forever hold onto that hope. I do believe that in my lifetime it will be regarded medically like the common cold, heart disease, diabetes or cancer.

The problem with the stigma, and the reason it's taking so long to kill it, is that we're not talking about decades worth. We're talking about centuries worth. Mental illness . . . that's a whole different problem. That's how people think. Sufferers used to be locked up in institutions and left to rot, thrown in the river, given up on. There was no hope back then. There is now.

36 The emotional cost of mental illness

I'm sure there are people out there that assume it was easy for me to 'come out' about my mental health issues. It wasn't easy, but ultimately I didn't have a choice, because I realised that when you keep the lid on these challenges it takes up a massive amount of your life energy. It's stressful and draining, and forces people to hide whole parts of themselves. This is happening each and every day in thousands of households across the country. And yet contrary to all the views we have of those suffering these disorders, often they're contributing to the community in amazing ways. When I read this letter I only wished we could make it easier for people to be honest about where they're at.

Thirty years ago I was diagnosed by a psychiatrist as suffering from manic depression—now bipolar disorder. For the 30 years preceding this I was regarded as a child, young person and adult who had a bad temper and who was extremely aggressive and overwhelming. At the time of diagnosis my marriage to a gambler/alcoholic had ended in divorce and I was with my to-be second husband. He supported me for twenty years but simultaneously used my disorder as a means of control and power. I have now been alone for twelve years. I have taken lithium for 30 years and am unable to survive without it. I have a number of uni degrees and am prominent in the community.

I spend a great deal of time with young people. I long to be able to share my situation with someone. I have tried with my family, whose answer was, 'It doesn't come from my side of the family!' My very favourite cousin died last year and he had been diagnosed many years before. He led a tortured existence. My dad had definite signs, as did another cousin. I have a daughter, a high achiever, for whom I agonise and look constantly for signs in. I have a full life, but an often lonely life. I wish I had the courage to 'go public' like you and declare who and what I am in the hope that things that happen to me and my behaviour—at times—would be understood, accepted and forgiven. But I am scared I would lose what I have. So everything remains a secret.

> Start by telling one person, someone you can trust and lean on. The relief will be overwhelming and will make it easier to tell more people.

Mental illness challenges relationships. It most definitely threatened my marriage. I would not have blamed Louise for walking away. It's particularly difficult before, or in the early stages of, diagnosis. Neither person properly grasps what they're really dealing with. Certain behavioural issues and mood swings seem impossible to understand. The shock to the system is real.

A lot of relationships are beyond repair at that point—and it's not until afterwards, when a diagnosis is delivered, that understanding arrives. It can be too late by then. The family is long gone, the relationship broken. As for keeping it a secret, I recommend coming clean. Start by telling one person, someone you can trust and lean on. The relief will be overwhelming and will make it easier to tell more people. If a friend rejects you because of it, they weren't worth your friendship anyway.

37 Soul mates

As far as I'm concerned soul mates are an indispensible part of surviving bipolar, but what do I mean by a soul mate? We get brainwashed into thinking that soul mates are two divinely linked creatures who magically form a blissfully harmonious existence that never cracks. From the moment they meet, they never say a bad word to each other, never feel or cause disappointment, never face hardships, never so much as roll their eyes at each other, never let each other down. Soul mates have two hearts beating as one.

Here's what I say to that: what a load of garbage! It's just an impossible ideal to strive for: you can never live up to all that yourself, and it's grossly unfair to lump that kind of expectation on your partner. It will end in heartache if that's what you're chasing because no-one can become what is an illusion in the first place. We see it in Hollywood movies, cartoons, Mills and Boon fiction, and music clips, and want it in our real lives, forgetting all those creations are pure fantasy.

I do believe in 'soul mates', however, 100 per cent. I also believe we have more than one. These are people who are special in your life and help you grow, whether you realise it or not. I'm living with mine. I just don't buy the magic carpet ride. You don't need to be giggling like teenagers all the time to be in a fantastic relationship.

Every couple has a honeymoon period and that's great, but no honeymoon can last the decades it takes to spend a lifetime together. The high divorce rate these days, one in three couples calling it quits, is sad—and has much to do with the impossible ideals we're chasing. Unrealistic expectations cause frustration and frustrations cause break-ups. The first minor tiff can feel like the end of the world. The illusion of everything being shiny forever is broken with the first disagreement.

People think that means they no longer have the perfect partner, or the bond has been broken for all time, so the union is on its way to ending. Louise and I have times when we fight like cat and dog, but there's nothing wrong with that because I have no doubt in my mind that she's my soul mate.

> 'Man is a knot into which relationships are tied.'
> Antoine de Saint-Exupéry

There's no shame in admitting we have our moments. We've had some BIG moments! It's perfectly normal. We're two human beings raising a family, living under the same roof—living in each other's pockets a lot of the time—and facing all the challenges of everyday life, and there are times when we drive each other stark, raving mad. But I love her. Show me a couple who reckon they don't have ups and downs and I'll show you a couple of liars.

Marriage can be bloody hard work—then throw mental illness into the mix. When I see my bipolar from Louise's point of view, the absolute shock to her system, the complete upheaval to her life, I'm overwhelmed. I very much doubt that as a little girl she dreamed of finding a handsome prince she'd end up having to repeatedly take to a psychiatric ward.

Louise could have done a runner during the hardest times and to be honest, I wouldn't have blamed her in the slightest. Why didn't she leave? I believe it's because there's genuine love between us, warts and all. We have stages of getting on each other's nerves but underneath all that is an understanding that we're in this for the long haul. That's just our deal.

> That is a soul mate: someone who rolls up their sleeves and helps in the hardest times.

I think about what Louise has done for me: every time the walls have come crashing down, every single time, Louise has been the first person by my side. She's found a way to have the kids looked after, cleared the decks at work or whatever else she had planned, because without a moment's hesitation, no questions asked, she's unfailingly dropped everything to come and help me. There's been nothing glamorous about it, but she's done it nonetheless. *That* is a soul mate: someone who rolls up their sleeves and helps in the hardest times. *That* is what I will take any day of the week.

The couples who try so hard to be shiny and perfect in public— please. No-one really knows what happens behind closed doors, but I'm guessing there isn't a single couple in the world going through life like Cinderella and her prince. I just don't buy it. Give me something real and unbreakable. Give me Louise. We push each other's buttons and it helps us grow.

I need someone to push me in the right direction. I don't want apathy in a relationship, where the air has been sucked out and we're staring out the window thinking, well, I guess we're stuck with each other now. Boredom isn't exactly a problem in our household. I don't want a relationship to *endure*. I want both of us to be on our toes. Be careful what you wish for! Apathy is worse than an occasional twelve-round bout of bickering.

Don't get me wrong. Louise and I aren't throwing plates at each other in the kitchen every night, either. Far from it: we get on like wildfire. But things pop up. You know, *things*. It's like a parent getting frustrated with the kids for watching too much TV. His frustration really stems from knowing they're capable of so much more. We all get frustrated in some of our family roles because we care enough to want the best.

Louise and I want our kids to have their own personalities, ideas, interests and lives. To chase their own dreams. Of course we do. Part of me wants to shape them into what I want them to be, but I also want to cut them enough slack so they can make a million mistakes, learn from those million mistakes, and move on. Kids and young adults need to be given the chance to develop at their own time and pace. Same goes with a marriage. I don't want two hearts beating as one. I want my own heart, and I want Louise to have hers.

Individuality is beautiful. It's just not humanly possible for two people to be on the same wavelength every minute of every day. There's too much pressure if that's the aim; too much pressure to even contemplate. Louise and I have talked about that a lot. I realise how lost I would have been without her, though. I'm not even sure I would still be alive. The most remarkable thing about Louise is this: everything she has done for me, she would have done for anyone. *That* is the kind of person she is.

She was right to call the police to Broadmeadow train station. She got to the Anzac Day car crash. She was in Sydney two hours after St Francis of Assisi made his telephone call. Serious, major stuff. What an incredible thing, for someone to care enough to be there every single time you need them. And for it to be no surprise at all when they do come through. There she is. Of course she is.

Afterwards, when I'm trying to sift through the wreckage of another episode, Louise has always been the difference between a decent ending and outright calamity. If she didn't call the police at Broadmeadow, if I'd actually boarded that train—there's no way of knowing what might have happened. If she hadn't arrived in Sydney so quickly—I shudder to think. She gets into her nursing mode. Methodical and efficient. Louise has helped me more than Dr Weiss. She's the one at the coalface, *all* the time.

Soul mates: teenagers think they'll find someone who'll make sure there's no bumps, bruises or bitchiness till death do they part. Don't be so unfair on the relationship to want that. Don't be so unfair on yourself. At some stage, you're both going to want to rip each other's heads off. Learn to deal with it.

We see the mirage of these allegedly perfect couples in cinemas, and on TV screens and magazine spreads with their million-dollar smiles and impossibly beautiful children, and we feel as if we don't measure up—we must be doing something wrong. That's a dangerous way of thinking.

Your soul mate might get a bit of food stuck between their teeth. Heaven forbid, they might even snore or put on a few kilos when they get older. Where does that leave you? Leave them be: you're probably not so perfect yourself. We think there can't be bad days, can't be arguments, because arguing means the love is gone. Wrong, wrong, wrong. I really don't want to be high and mighty enough to say that most people's image of soul mates is a crock. I really don't want to sound that crude. But it's a crock.

The good times will always be there. You wouldn't have started dating and gone down the aisle otherwise. Don't blow the bad times out of proportion. People say, 'When I find my soul mate, we'll never argue with each other. It will be all just perfect because we'll have meant to be together.' Well, I hate to rain on the parade, but through experience, I know your true soul mate in life is also the person who can frustrate you the most.

Your soul mate can argue with you, disappoint you, not always share the values you have. You can misunderstand each other, confuse each other—all of these things are true of Louise and me. Both ways. But here's the thing: at the end of the day, the commitment is unconditional and mutual. Louise does not sugar-coat anything. When I'm being a pain in the backside, depression or not, she will tell me so. But she has shown her commitment time and again. She could have told me, with complete justification, that I wasn't the same man she married and she wanted me out. I know she's thought it and I'm fine with that. That's reality.

In our own ways we've evolved and grown and matured and developed into the best people we can be from all the pushing, cajoling, massaging and shoving we've given each other. Mostly it's been for my own good even when I haven't realised it at the time. In the big picture, that's what soul mates do for each other. They help. They become two gloriously independent people who are always on each other's side.

We've been together a long time. I was seventeen and Louise was sixteen when we first met. That was more than 30 years ago. We had a connection straight away. We shake our heads at being together longer than we've been apart in our lifetimes. I make fun of it, but think it's brilliant. We're both in our late 40s and it's staggering to think we've spent our entire adult lives together. We look at each other and wonder where the time has gone. We've grown up side by side—and believe me, there have been times when it's been a rough old ride. I'm actually quite difficult to live with at times. There's a revelation!

Everything I've talked about here, the good and the bad, describes my relationship with Louise. The wheels fell off when I was diagnosed. Many relationships don't survive that kind of earthquake to the system, but Louise and I are living proof it can be done. I do get why it can be terminal to the marriage. It can be just too traumatic, too much of a shock, too hot to handle.

There's a great song by Bon Iver about being patient, about being kind. Don't do anything rash. The fact Louise stayed, and she did so much to keep the marriage together through all the challenges of the past decade, proves a relationship doesn't have to be endless smooth sailing to be a triumph. We're human beings. Even if it's not always pretty, a marriage is worth clinging to as long as you can.

My trouble is that I can get a bit flippant about it. After an episode I tend to dust myself off, consign it to ancient history and move on. But when I look at what's happened in the last twelve years, there's been some absolutely huge issues for us to get through, and times when I've taken Louise's selflessness for granted. I recognise clearly how enormous some of the predicaments have been, and how Louise has been the saviour. I've let her down a lot more than she's let me down. In fact, I don't think she's ever let me down with anything important.

After the Craig-dominated lunch with friends in March 2010, my pulse was racing off the scale by four o'clock and I was becoming delusional. Louise recognised all the signs, put me in the car and took me straight up to James Fletcher. Again I was admitted before any damage was done; again she was the one to take control. That, to me, is a soul mate. When the chips are down and I desperately need someone to step in, Louise is there.

Words can be nice but they're also too easy. You'll know your soul mate through their actions. You can say whatever you like to your partner, make every promise under the sun, but the nitty gritty is about being there in times of crisis. Every couple needs romance, but they've also got to fight on each other's behalf. Big things, little things—Louise really would have done it for anyone. What a truly amazing thing that is. What she's done for me, I'm not entirely sure I could have done for her. Does that sound callous?

I've told Louise. She understands. After the first time at the train station, after we'd been through the whole gruelling recovery from depression, our whole lives were turned upside down. When we didn't know what the hell was going on Louise basically nursed me through while still having the kids and her own career and the run of the household to manage. When she supported me every minute of every day while I was at my lowest ebb, seriously wondering if life was even worth living, I got very emotional about it and said: 'I don't know if I could be this strong for you. I just don't know if I could do what you're doing.'

Her commitment, compassion and selflessness completely blows me away. They're admirable and inspiring. Actually I think I could do it for Louise now, but only because she's shown me how. She can be the most stubborn, frustrating and annoying woman I know—and I love her dearly.

38 Louise's take on things

I've talked a lot about Louise throughout the book, so now it's time for her slant on things.

To say Craig and I are on a learning curve is an understatement. There have been more episodes in the last seven years than the first five, when there was only the one, really, at Broadmeadow in 2000. Craig becomes unwell, we get through it, we try to learn from it for next time, life goes back to normal for a while but then another episode comes. That's the cycle we're in. I think to myself: Why has it come again? We've done this right; we've made sure of this, that and the other. We've done everything we can to make sure Craig's had enough rest.

We try to make sure life isn't too stressful but Craig is pegging out again. I think: Is there something we're missing? Am I doing something wrong? Is there something else we both need to be doing? But I don't beat myself up about it any more. There doesn't need to be a reason for an episode, it's just the way it is. At Craig's stage and age, bipolar can just get a bit cranky and irritable, no matter what we do.

The nature of Craig's highs is different. He used to have quite a reasonable and predictable build-up to an elevation, maybe over a week or two. There would be very clear signs of what was coming. That's changed. The warnings aren't as obvious. He can become psychotic in a very short period of time.

> 'Love is temporary insanity curable by marriage.'
>
> Ambrose Bierce

On the last occasion, after that football game at Parramatta in 2010, it took only a few hours for the high to hit. Back then, if we could nail it on the way up, if I could talk him into going to hospital, we could put a lid on it in time. If we missed that window of opportunity, that's when the police and everyone else would have to be involved.

I think Craig's bipolar has learned how to run a bit faster now. After that lunch described in the chapter 'The Black Dog comes back', when he was back here at home, one minute he was actually quite OK, but the next he was away. He's had so many episodes that sometimes they just blend into one when I start thinking about them. We both learn something from each experience. The biggest one I've learned is that he has to look after himself. It's taken me this long to realise I can only do so much.

Craig is the one who has to take ownership of it. He's the one who has to self-evaluate and take steps to stay healthy. He's the one who has to monitor his medication. He's the only one who can do it. Other people can help him, and that's important, but we can't be his be-all and end-all. If he's feeling too up, he's the one who has to pull himself down.

> 'Craig has to look after himself. It's taken me this long
> to realise I can only do so much.'
>
> Louise

'I refuse to buy into Craig's depressions. I can't afford to.'

Louise

When he manages that part of it, we don't end up with the highs; we don't end up with the psychosis; we don't end up with the depression; we don't end up with anything we cannot manage. Home isn't disrupted and life carries on. To me, from when Craig is unwell to when he's better, from when he's psychotic to being back to normal, it's a good twelve months. It really is that long. There's an episode, he's in hospital for a week or two, he comes home—but he's still not quite properly well. There's a couple more weeks of the initial episode hanging round like a bad smell, he might be well-ish for a week or two—and then we have the depression, which can take months. Only after he comes through the depression is he completely well again and I really do think it's a whole year from start to finish.

I refuse to buy into his depressions. I can't afford to. I don't have the energy, so I've made myself immune. It used to be different. I'd get dragged down by it and worry whether Craig was eating enough, drinking enough fluids. I'd be fretting about him getting out of bed and moving around, making sure every last little thing was right. But then I thought: *Stuff this*. I told him: 'This is your problem. This is what happens, you have your highs and this is your payback. It's not nice, it's ugly, but I cannot deal with it and bail you out.

'I've got a house to run, we've got three kids, I've got a job, I need to concentrate on them. I'm really sorry but I'm not going to get thrown off by your depression. You know I'm here for you, but it's *your* depression. I'm not going to waste all my energy on you. I need it for too many other things.'

It probably doesn't sound very nice but I think it's helped Craig realise the condition is his. I used to mollycoddle him too much.

Now, when he's depressed, I don't really care. Well, of course I care, but I can't help him half as much as he can help himself. Yes, it can be a pain in the neck: We'll be invited out but we can't go because Craig is depressed. That's fine, I often go anyway. Not to anything where there will be strangers but to family functions, somewhere I know friends will be, I'll turn up and have a great time. I used to stay home, but not any more. I tell whoever it is that Craig's depressed, he can't come—years ago, I never said anything but it's no big deal now. I'll go to something alone and someone will say, 'Craig unwell?' I'll say, 'Yep', and that's that. It's all anyone needs to know. If we started telling lies, a few fibs to keep it in-house, we'd never be able to keep it up anyway because the depression is going to last quite a few months.

Even just three months of cover-ups, that's too much hard work. I'd rather just spit out the truth. Other people are more into keeping skeletons in cupboards and never telling anyone anything about themselves. That's fine; it's different for different people. We've all got skeletons, we've all got secrets in the cupboard. Some cupboards are just bigger than others. Some people have wardrobes full of skeletons, some people just have one little drawer, but we all have them. I've got no interest in hiding anything.

For some reason, even before Craig was diagnosed, I never had a problem dealing with mental health issues. I've always understood how real it is. I've only ever been a medical nurse: heart attacks, strokes, pneumonia. I haven't done any psychiatric work but with patients affected by drugs and alcohol, mental health issues come up that you have to deal with on the run. Even with general patients, there's a lot of psych out there to be learned on the job.

As much as I get it, I've also seen that a lot of people, nurses included, do not. They just do not like the issue of mental health, period. It makes them very uncomfortable. Even before it started applying to Craig, I was: 'Righto, someone is a patient here, this is how they feel, they obviously can't help it, let's work out what we can do for them.'

Since Craig was diagnosed I've come to know a lot about it. I tell the doctors; you've got to be really careful with this drug, add some of this, they look at me and say, 'Are you a psych nurse? Because you should be.' I tell them I only have some knowledge because my husband has mental health issues. I can see them thinking: *Sorry I asked.*

'I'm not going to sugar-coat it. This is hard work.'

Louise

People can have very narrow views. Don't get me wrong, I'm not the most worldly person, either, but in my line of work, nursing, you do see all kinds. I think that gives me a bigger tolerance and understanding of what's out there. I'm not going to sugar-coat it. This is hard work. It's been twelve years now and I'm used to it being part of our life. We had a bit of a false start: we had the explosion at Broadmeadow but then there was a nice honeymoon period of about five years. Everything seemed normal again. I thought OK, Craig has this condition, but life's not much different. There were changes—Craig found God, he changed his outlook on life, he got rid of alcohol, he changed quite a few things—but there weren't any upsets or disruptions at home for those first five years. Life went on. But then he started to become unwell, regularly. That's when it felt like the bipolar had really moved in with us. So this was what life was really going to be like.

Some people get cancer, some people have heart troubles,

Craig just happened to be lumped with this. The important thing is that we have periods of him being well. Without that, to be honest, I might be thinking, is this worth it? But because we do have so many good periods, and we know he can be well for twelve to eighteen months at a time, we've got that time to recuperate and reorganise. We get the old Craig and our old lives back even though the bipolar will probably start up again at some stage. That's just the way it is, and that's OK. Whatever comes up, we'll deal with it.

He doesn't remember most of what happened after that football game at Parramatta in 2010. I'll fill in the gaps for him. We knocked him out pretty good. Straight after he called from his hotel, I was on the phone to my friend Kim: 'We've got another episode. I need someone to come with me to Sydney because I don't know what I'm going to find when I get there. I don't know what I'm walking into.' The hardest thing is getting the phone call: here we go again. I'm crying when I think about this—I don't know why, I should be past that by now . . . anyway, as Craig said earlier, Kim came with me.

I did need some back-up and she's a trained nurse, too. It can take more than one person to contain Craig when he's running wild. I might need Kim to make calls, do whatever needs to be done behind the scenes. I've probably only driven to Sydney five times in my life and Craig couldn't tell me the address of the hotel. He just vaguely said, 'It's the same place I've always been to.' I'd only been there once. I drove over the Harbour Bridge— thankfully it was a Sunday morning so there wasn't really any traffic. Twenty-four hours later would have been a nightmare. It was 7 a.m. when we got to Sydney. We looked up and I said to Kim, see that building there, that's the one we want. 'If I'm turning and we're getting further from that building, tell me!'

Well, we eventually got there, went in, did what we had to. Craig actually looked a lot better than I thought he would.

But when I sat down and talked to him, there was still a bit of madness there, I could see it in his eyes. The 'mad cow' look, I call it. I'd brought an antipsychotic drug with me, Risperidone. I said to Kim: 'How much do you reckon we give him, two or four?' She said: 'Let's just slog him with four.' I said, 'Yep, sounds good to me!'

We sat there for probably half an hour and he still wasn't coming down. I thought the drugs weren't going to work. We couldn't get to Newcastle in the state he was in. It's nearly a two-and-a-half hour trip and he'd probably jump out of the car or grab the steering wheel or something crazy like that. It'd be too dangerous to be doing a 100 kilometres an hour on the freeway with him in the back seat. So we had to take him to the nearest hospital.

We took him to the emergency department of the RPA. They told us it was going to be a 45-minute wait. Craig started sweating, looking like crap and saying he didn't feel well. Kim and I were trying to hold him up, he was flopping round—it was dreadful. Being nurses, we had no sympathy. We were actually propping him up so if he did fall, he'd go headfirst because then the nurses would have to come and look at him. If he slid sideways off the chair, or just slumped onto us, they could keep ignoring him. If he went down, we wanted him going flat on his face. That was the nurse coming out in us—tricks of the trade.

He started to get really drowsy when the drugs took hold. I went to the nurse and said, 'Remind me how long Risperidone lasts? I think it's got a really long half-life.'

We looked it up on her computer.

'You've got twelve hours before he needs another dose,' she said.

'Right, we're out of here, I'm taking him back to Newcastle, we can sort it out there,' I told her. We grabbed a wheelchair, threw Craig in it, still not much sympathy—the nurse said, 'Love your work, girls.' She was my kind of age, an old nurse who thought, Yep, go on, chuck him in the back seat and off you go. I knew Craig would rather be in Newcastle than Sydney when he came to.

He slept the whole way, other than for a few words. He was almost comatose, actually. One of my other girlfriends asked me, Weren't you worried about his airway? Short answer: no. I wasn't worried about frigging anything! All I cared about was getting down that freeway and getting home. I was more worried driving *to* Sydney, not knowing how bad he was, than on the trip back.

Every episode we had before then, there had been huge drama, the police and whatnot. (The time the cops came to our house after Craig's lunch: they were actually of no help at all. They didn't know what to do. They're a bit of muscle power but they're just not trained in how to handle mental health. We've done it twice, calling the police, but I'll try not to do it again because they're really more of a hindrance.) We drove back up to Newcastle and put him in James Fletcher. 'Well,' they said, 'you've definitely got enough drugs into him.'

I know my nursing background is a blessing. I've nursed my whole life, and I've looked after people who are psychotic when I've been in the drug and alcohol units. I've worked with a lot of people with dementia, nothing surprises me too much. Craig's right when he says I go into nurse mode. I find the more unwell people get, the calmer I am. That's the nursing training. It's a learned skill. If I'm not calm, if I'm wigging out when I'm supposed to be the one helping, what hope is there for anyone else? I can yell and scream with the best of them in general life. I can rant and rave; I can do all those things, but most things don't bother me too much.

When there's a big situation, I get into professional mode, and that's how I cope with Craig's episodes. There are good points to having the training: yes, I know what to do, I know where to take him, I know the hospital system, I know when things aren't working and what channels to go through. My background is a blessing for those reasons, but there are some non-blessings, too. On the drive to Sydney, for example, I'm anticipating all the scenarios I might find, because I've seen how bad it can be. I probably waste a bit of energy on worrying and making plans for things I don't even know will happen.

When Craig had his first episode in 2000, I thought, Oh my God, what is going on here? I knew it was really odd and bizarre but I was already so worn out, trying to keep everything together at home, that I didn't really have the energy to sit down and think, why is he doing this? And then when the doctors told me what it was I thought, Well, that adds up, doesn't it? A lot of things added up.

I can be mentally and emotionally exhausted when Craig is going through the mania–depression cycle but, again, we get through. It can take *me* six months to feel good again. I still get everything done, I hope, but the tiredness can wear me down. That's life. Everyone has their problems to deal with. We have our battles, too, but the history between us helps.

We were married for thirteen or fourteen years before the bipolar came along. When you have history like we do, you know it's worth working hard to save the marriage. I can imagine without that, it would be easier to say, 'You know what? This is too hard.' I can completely see why a lot of couples might not survive it. Why the other partner would say: this isn't what I bought into. But when you've got a strong background, you *want* to put in the work. I know the real Craig so I just wait for this other version to go away. I know what he's really like.

We had fourteen years of good. We're having a bit of a hiccup in the cycle of being married, but I can handle that. There are definitely times when I think the cycle has taken us too far the other way, especially if the hiccups are a bit close together, but I'm not going anywhere. A mental health issue in a relationship definitely tests how much love there is, whether you think it's worth your while. You can only stay if you can see a potential for happiness. I think we're doing great—but the money is a concern.

> 'We're having a bit of a hiccup in the cycle of being married, but I can handle that.'
>
> Louise

I think mental health is the way it is because a lot of people can't afford good psychiatry. The cost of appointments adds up fast. The stress of that can make things worse. Doing that regularly, and this doesn't include the cost of medications that are not on the PBS, can be a strain. But Craig's psychiatrist, Dr Weiss, is brilliant and worth every cent. He's fantastic at tweaking and finetuning medications, he seems to have this fantastic knowledge of what needs to be done. He's kept Craig well most of the time.

Craig is more on top of it now than ever. A few years ago, he wouldn't listen to anyone about the high. It was like taking a little kid to Luna Park: he's having the time of his life but then I have to grab his hand and tell him he has to leave—for his own good. When Craig is elevating, when he's in his Luna Park, he thinks it's the greatest thing that has ever happened to him. I'm trying to tell him it *isn't* good—this is actually really bad for you. He's like, oh piss off! You don't know what you're talking about! Let me have some fun! I have to pick that window of opportunity when he's getting higher and higher, but still rational enough to listen. When he'll still take his medication or let me take him to hospital. That's the trick, but one we don't always get right.

'It was like taking a little kid to Luna Park: he's having the time of his life but then I have to grab his hand and tell him he has to leave—for his own good.'

Louise

His talks cause angst between us: I say, 'No, you're travelling too far, it's too many days away from home, you know the deal: one a month is OK, two a month if it's in Newcastle. You want to do it to help people and that's fine, but you also have to make sure you're staying well yourself.' I'm proud of him for doing it. He'll come home saying, 'Louise, what a great night! I met the most amazing people! You won't believe their stories!' He really is interested in every person there. I've seen him work a room, saying hello to everyone, asking them about their lives: none of it is an act, he really is interested. I can think of nothing worse than going with him, getting cornered by people I don't know and bombarded with questions. I'm proud of Craig for being so open about his life, but I have reservations about him writing this book. Not because I don't want people to know, more because I fear the impact it might have on him.

The pressure of writing it, the deadline to get it done, the book signings and interviews and promotional work afterwards: it's all pretty hectic. All that activity can lead to more episodes. It has nothing to do with preferring to keep it a secret. I've never cared if the whole world knows. In Newcastle, basically three-quarters of the people have known from the start anyway. He's on the radio; everyone knows him—and there aren't many secrets in this town at the best of times. I'm just worried about whether he can stay well after the book is published. We'll have to watch him then.

Part of me thinks, Craig, do we really need this? Do we really need it in our lives? I could have put my foot down and said no, but he was going to do it anyway so there was no point. I do think it's wonderful that a person can get up on a stage in front of an audience of hundreds to put a positive view across about mental health and educate people. I think it very much needs doing and I'm glad he feels that calling. Apparently he talks very well. Apparently a lot of people get a lot of worth out of what he says. The main thing is that he's doing it for the right reasons. Would I want to do it? Not on your life! It's just not who I am. I'll sit down with two or three people and tell them every-thing . . . these are the things I do, this helps, and so on . . . I'm comfortable in small gatherings but I cannot do the stage.

I talk to people in hospital wards. I have friends over. Once, a woman called and asked if she could come around for a coffee. She turned up and said, 'My husband's depressed and I just want to know how you survive because I don't know if I can do it.' She said *she* was the one going insane. I told her I knew what she meant: when they're depressed, they stand next to you, right on your shoulder, sucking the bejesus out of you, draining all your energy. They follow you around, telling you the same story over and over and over until you want to headbutt them. Then they want to sleep all the time and don't want to talk to you. She said, 'You've just described my husband.'

I said, 'Actually, I've actually just described depression.' That's what it's like for everyone. I could see how relieved she was. I told her it's miserable and hard work. When it's severe, you can't leave them too often because you're not quite sure they're well enough to be left alone. But you get to the point where you've had enough of them and if you don't get out of the house, you'll be the one who ends up in hospital from exhaustion, and then what happens to the household? I told her to just accept it as a balancing act.

Talk to your friends, I said. Don't keep secrets. Don't pretend you're coping when you're not. Little things like taking multi-vitamins, I think that's important because you get so stressed, and spend so much time running around looking after everybody else, that you forget about your own wellbeing. Everyone says, 'How's Craig?' Sometimes I feel like saying, 'Stuff Craig, anyone care how I'm going?' Don't do any more than you have to. Pay the bills, look after the kids, concentrate on the basics. I told her your social life will be diminished but that'll be OK because you won't have the energy to go out anyway.

> 'Talk to your friends. Don't keep secrets. Don't pretend you're coping when you're not.'
>
> Louise

Have someone you like or trust, someone who's a good adviser, and lean on them as much as you have to. Don't be ashamed of reaching out for their support. When you're really, really pulling your hair out, ring your friend and put your foot down: 'We're talking about *this* today whether you want to or not!' Get it out of your system.

Let's not pretend it's fun. When they become well, you need to take some time to recover, too. That's easy to overlook. Never be too hard on yourself. It's easy to think you're not doing enough when really, things can be out of your control. I told the woman that I monitor Craig's medication when he's really, really unwell because he can't even remember if he's taken his drugs. I'm onto that. But once he's getting better, it's his problem. Feed him, water him, get him to bed, I say.

A friend whose husband has the same condition gets physically aggressive, he'll start throwing punches—that would be frightening. Craig isn't aggressive, ever. I might not be able to reason with him. I might not be able to get him to do what I want, but he's never physically abusive. He's been verbally aggressive, very forceful in what he's saying to other people, but never verbally abusive to me. He'll swear like a trucker but none of it makes me feel in any danger at all. I don't think Craig's capable of that. It's just not in his nature. Craig is on a noble cause when he's high. It's just that nobody else, including me, knows what the cause is. He's just trying to save the world! A lot of us, all of us, get elevated moods. We're happy and we love it. But Craig's moods tip really quickly into mania. That's when I get narky with him: you've put too much on your plate, this is a recipe for disaster.

My understanding of it is that there's a little button in our brains that Craig is without. We all get a bit overexcited and hyperactive. When the rest of us have been going a million miles an hour for a couple of days and we just can't do it any more, we stop, exhausted. We know when enough is enough. We go and sit at home for 24 hours and relax. But when Craig gets to that point, that's when he pings and flies to the next stage. There doesn't seem to be the button in his brain that says 'Stop'.

Every time he becomes psychotic, part of me is saying: Oh no, here we go again. It's not so much the psychosis, because once I get him to hospital I know he's safe. It's getting him there that can be such hard work. If we miscue it, we're up the creek and it's nothing but headbutting. It's getting the police involved, it's getting thrown in the back of paddy wagons, it's getting the kids organised so they don't see too much of it. That's the worst, but once he's in hospital, they've got control of it; he's locked up and safe. That's the easy bit.

I don't visit him every day. Only every second or third. It's my time to sort things out at home, get the house organised. He's going to be unwell for a while and we'll have a few more hoops to jump through. The kids are very good through these periods. They all stick around him pretty closely, keeping an eye on him, it's nice. They don't tease him like they would normally do when Craig is feeling well; they're very careful. They don't engage Craig as much, mainly because he doesn't want to be engaged. They give him space because he needs it.

Every family has issues to get through. I'm glad we just tell them the truth. They take in what they need. They can see what's happening. We don't play games in this house. Don't call a mental health issue something it isn't. Give kids enough information to satisfy their curiosity: don't go overboard, but don't lie and don't tell them something you know is wrong because it will find a way to come back and bite you.

> 'Give kids enough information to satisfy their curiosity.'
>
> Louise

Life is great at the moment, really, really great. It's nice to have Craig well for a long period. I think he gets it now: he has an illness but there are steps he can take to keep himself well. He knows he has to take his pills, see his doctor, exercise, eat well, have a low alcohol intake and try to make life as stress-free as possible. The main thing I want to tell anyone reading this: there's light at the end of the tunnel. Right now, Craig is the most consistently well he's been in the last five years. It's nice to see.

The last time he was elevating, I did have to take him to hospital, but only because I didn't have any drugs in the house. Now I have a cupboard full, and I know what to do. Dr Weiss has him on a couple of new drugs that really seem to be doing the trick. Craig has more insight and acceptance. The realisation has clicked that if he doesn't have the highs, he doesn't have the lows, and a person like Craig fears the lows more than anything. It's like your alcoholic. They hit rock bottom but they have to be the ones, and only them, to decide they're never going to drink again. Craig needed to decide that he didn't want the highs. He hates the depressions. He doesn't cope well with them.

He's a pain in the frigging backside when he's depressed, just this misery hanging around the house. He's harder work when he's depressed because the depressions last longer. He doesn't go anywhere, he doesn't do anything, he doesn't go out, he just locks himself into a room or hangs around the house, driving me nuts most of the time, but at least I know where he is. When he's psychotic, I don't know what he's doing, and that's the scary part. He could be totally out of control. The other thing is sometimes people never get out of the high. Every time you have a psychotic episode, you're doing damage, and it can get to the point where the damage is irreversible. Recovery from an episode can't be taken for granted. There's always the chance, and the little fear in the back of my head, that Craig won't ever come out of a psychosis. The great lesson in all of this is simply take each day as it comes . . . tomorrow arrives quick enough!

39 Vivid lifetime memories

I now realise I am just one small piece of the universal puzzle. My struggles and triumphs are no more severe or important than anyone else's. We're all on the same planet. We're all part of history's march. I can remember where I was and what I was doing for every landmark event of our time. It helps me understand what an amazing world this is. How lucky I am to be here.

> I think there's great benefit in looking back over your life and seeing what a mind-blowing journey it all is.

The significant moments in history are so clear to me. I know where I was when I was six and when Neil Armstrong walked on the moon, and when the 'Thriller in Manila' was fought between Muhammad Ali and Joe Frazier in 1975. I remember exactly where I was when I heard the news that John Lennon was shot and, the following year, when Dennis Lillee broke Lance Gibbs' world record for Test wickets in cricket. I can remember where I was when Australia won sailing's America's Cup. And I can remember the first day I saw Louise.

I think there's great benefit in looking back over your life and seeing what a mind-blowing journey it all is. We're part of it, too, just by being alive at this time. We've already had amazing experiences, good and bad, no matter how old we are. So many mundane things pass us by but some events, like when your children are born, when you propose to your wife, when you see her walking down the aisle, when someone close to you dies— those events are significant and they're part of all our stories.

I'm still opening my eyes to the history unfolding round me every day. There's that old Chinese saying: 'May you live in interesting times.' We do! I don't believe it for one moment when someone says life was so much better in the good old days. It's a myth, a fallacy . . . How brilliantly fascinating is the world right now. I look back and think, wow, in my lifetime I've seen man walk on the moon. I think about people who were around in 1903: Orville and Wilbur Wright got an aeroplane off the ground despite people saying it could never happen. Just 60 years after that—just an instant in history—we're on the moon. That's mind-boggling to me. Now we're talking about a manned mission to Mars! Whether you and I are around long enough to see it, it will happen. Incredible. It's fascinating to track the human race and it ensures I don't get bogged down in my own world. It's why I accept my place in the unfurling story of seven billion people: what I have and who I am.

What I have is bipolar 1 disorder. What I am is a man trying to make the best of his life in a big, bustling world. I think I'm going alright, but I want an expert opinion. I want Dr Weiss's verdict: Alan has been my doctor since early 2001. Since then he has guided the ship very skilfully, at times through some fairly rough seas. I value his judgement and trust it completely.

40 My doc lends his perspective

Having looked at so many aspects of living with mental issues, it would have been an oversight not to include my good doctor as well.

Craig thought it was all over in 2005. He thought he was cured. He'd been through depression on the other side of mania from Broadmeadow, he'd written a book and thought that was the end of it. I wanted him to acknowledge there was a lot more work to be done, and he did, but deep down he thought that he had done it, he had beaten bipolar. That was reflected in his eagerness to get off medication and try alternative treatments, which I'm not against: alternative treatments have their place but, as we've seen in Craig's past five years, they don't do enough on their own.

He's had three manic episodes, and at least three depressions, one of which lasted nine months and was really severe. I think that last depression is what took the wind out of his sails. Craig had become non-compliant with his medication because he had gone a long period without an episode but the illness was still there, rumbling away in the background. I think he was surprised by the strength of its return. Not on an intellectual level, because he knew he had an illness, but I think he was surprised by its force on an emotional level. It gave him another under-layer of insight.

If I had to summarise Craig's past five years, the advancement has been in the development of insight, a deeper understanding of how this terrible illness can get him. It's bad luck to have pneumonia, but you have treatment and you can get better. There's a different understanding needed here: the importance of treatment, but also the understanding you won't get completely better, ever. Craig won't get to the stage where bipolar just disappears.

With bipolar 2, with enough education and psychotherapy, which can be quite powerful, and lifestyle changes, it might be able to be managed very well. I had one woman with bipolar 2 disorder who went years without medication. She had the advantage of being very wealthy so she was able to dedicate herself to the management process without having to work. She could stay in the house if she was depressed, contain it if she felt a bit manic. But basically, bipolar doesn't leave.

Craig has two advantages: his marriage and his employer. Marriages often break down in these circumstances but to Louise's credit, she's hung in there. The ABC is clearly an understanding employer. I think having those two things gives Craig a better chance than a lot of other people. In other cases, I've seen a trail of manic episodes and the gradual decline of function. It escalates completely out of control.

Louise calls a spade a spade, which is what Craig needs. He's allowed me to have dialogue with her, another plus. I always know, if Louise is in the waiting room when Craig comes to see me, that something more sinister is going on. He'll bring Louise if there's a real issue swirling around—and he deserves credit for that. It's helped the three of us stay on the same page. I know what state Craig is in as soon as I greet him in the waiting room. It's very easy to pick when he's a bit high. When he's a bit low, he doesn't have that edge, he loses his sociability. When you get to know someone quite well, as I have with Craig over many years, you pick up the nuances of their personality. Craig knows that I know what's going on before he even tells me. Which I think is sometimes why he doesn't want to see me.

To explain bipolar to those unfamiliar: we all get high, but we don't get hypomanic-high. We can all feel euphoric when we have a 'cloud nine' experience. We're watching a sunset and that can be a really uplifting moment, but it's not even close to hypomania because we're still in control of our intellect. With bipolar, there's a switch that doesn't go off when it should.

When Craig is heading towards hypomania, there's an escalating series of symptoms, which include his thoughts speeding up, and his speech trying to match the pace of his thoughts but being unable to, which builds even more pressure—in severe mania you have the flight of ideas. Random thoughts come together too fast and he misses out on the connective information. Then he gets compulsive and loses perspective of what's right and wrong. Sound judgement disappears. Craig, as do all bipolar sufferers, becomes very grandiose.

The religious bent is a common theme in mania. I guess the most grandiose person that anyone can imagine is Jesus Christ. It's the ultimate altruistic act, isn't it, to do something fantastic for others, so religious imagery is always prevalent in the hypomanic state, which is where Craig has been. He's only very briefly touched mania because the medication has worked in time. Hypomania is below mania, but above normal. If we talk about level of function—and function revolves around work, social interaction, the family dynamic—we find that people can still be quite functional despite some hypomanic behaviour.

'The challenge is for Craig to really have the insight
that . . . even though he's having a lot of fun, he's
entering dangerous territory, he's probably doing too
much, he's being reckless.'

Dr Alan Weiss

My worry with Craig is when he gets busy with his football calling. The finals come around, the adrenaline rushes are cranked up and away he goes. Craig has become a sought after public speaker, and he does a fantastic job with *beyondblue* and those organisations, but it's another way the horse can bolt. When he's doing all these talks and going away a lot, when he's saying yes to everything and burning the candle at both ends, that brings up some real issues for us.

It's complex with Craig because it's not just his bipolar: he has a large personality style anyway. He's a radio announcer so he's got to be a bit grand, a bit narcissistic, otherwise he's not going to be a very good presenter. I think that's another component that can make his mania take off: that he's a bit like that anyway. He's a very likeable chap, he's everybody's mate; he's like that even when he's not manic. The challenge is for Craig to really have the insight that when he's in that state of plus-one or plus-two, what he does next could be really quite destructive. Even though he's having a lot of fun, he's entering dangerous territory: he's probably doing too much and he's being reckless.

People can ruin their careers and lives in mania, it really can be that destructive. Craig's alternative therapies are a good add-on as long as they in no way replace the traditional medicine approach. The baseline needs to be right, and medication is that baseline. That's what sets the foundation. The worry is that with all his alternative treatments, it's easy for that to become grandiose, for Craig to think he can treat himself without being aware he's hypomanic just thinking along those lines. Craig is definitely at risk of that. He's often talked me down when it comes to medication: we don't need that, it's time to get me off this. Not so much now, but in the early days he talked like this.

He knows now, however, that everything he does is important. His openness helps, the lack of shame or embarrassment. I had issues of stigma with a top athlete recently. He was worried what his teammates would think of him having a mental illness. We were able to work through it enough for him to tell his coach. He then told his teammates and received an overwhelmingly positive response. There was no stigma at all in what he thought might be an unforgiving environment.

People care, I've found. And it gives them an explanation for what has seemed like rather bizarre behaviour. That athlete had withdrawn from the team for a number of days due to being suicidally depressed. They were aware something odd was happening, so their relief to hear the real story was matched by the athlete's relief at having told it.

> 'The experience of the high . . . can be addictive to anyone.'
>
> Dr Alan Weiss

My concern is that Craig's personality is so closely linked to a tendency towards mania and that the fondness for the high will return. One of the most powerful shows I've seen in recent years is Stephen Fry's BBC series on bipolar. One of the things that stood out on that show (it didn't necessarily surprise me but it was striking) was that out of his whole bipolar group, I think only two people, when asked if they could be born with bipolar or without it, pushed the red button and said they wouldn't want it. All the rest would have it again. That's the grip that mania can take on people. That's where the worry is.

Craig can love the experience of the high. It can be addictive to anyone. Craig is being very creative now with this book, but I have a problem with how famous people with bipolar are presented. It's like a *60 Minutes* show. It's only a snapshot: two days of footage is condensed into a ten-minute segment. We don't get the full picture. The perception is that they're creative and brilliant because of their mania. But often when someone is in that hypomanic state, and they come back to what they've written, what they've done is really quite bad. No-one would seriously consider publishing it because it's not very good. What *they* think is good is distorted and they need to be on a more even keel to tidy it up. Craig right now is neither up nor down. I don't always need to see him to know how he's going.

I can switch into his mood simply by hearing him on the radio. From listening to his voice calling the footy or doing his Saturday morning show: I know exactly where he's at and what state he's in. Like I say, to be a good radio announcer he needs charisma: he's talking to himself, basically, and generally with great animation. When he's feeling off, he loses that. He loses the grand presentation.

If there's a downward spiral, he loses enthusiasm, he loses the will to do it and then he loses the idea that it's even worth doing at all. The ultimate retreat is into feeling so bad he thinks the world is better off without him. Craig has had those moments of feeling helpless but he has such a great network of people around him that the risks of the most unfortunate outcome are lessened. It's much harder for people on their own when they don't have a check-and-balance like Craig has with Louise.

He's gone without an episode now for more than a year. That's testament to his actions and willingness to do what needs to be done. It's been so long that I think he could enjoy quite a long period without a psychotic episode if we keep him balanced.

We've got the medication right, and he has the insight that what doesn't swing up doesn't swing down. He has made significant lifestyle changes and matured in his understanding of the illness. I would say that Craig has come of age.

41 The eleven commandments

We've covered a huge amount of ground here. If you were to ask me to put all I've learned in a nutshell, then here are my eleven commandments for a genuinely better life. To get you in the mood, I just have to quote Stacey Charter: 'Don't rely on someone else for your happiness and self-worth. Only you can be responsible for that. If you can't love and respect yourself—no-one else will be able to make that happen. Accept who you are—completely; the good and the bad—and make changes as YOU see fit—not because you think someone else wants you to be different.'

These are my must-haves for a better life with bipolar disorder:

1. Accept where you're at

Nothing productive happened until I accepted I had an illness. At first, disbelief played a part: I can't be bipolar. I can't be! Then I had to get over the idea that it could be conquered or simply disappear. I slipped into thinking maybe it wasn't really depression: I was just going through a rough patch, a midlife crisis; maybe everyone gets like this. Maybe my case is different from

everyone else's and this is just a one-off. I'm a sturdy bloke—
maybe I'm better equipped to beat it. I was flapping like I'd never
flapped before.

In the early days I fought it like Ali, but fighting was harder
than accepting. I fought it, I tried to hide from my depression,
I tried to keep it quiet for a little while until I realised the best I
could do was to surrender to it. That's when I did actually win
the fight. The relief was like cool, fresh water on my face.

My life had turned upside down, but nothing compared to
acceptance for impact and peace of mind. It took me years
to accept the realities. I thought I knew everything but I knew
nothing. I had to accept some hard home truths: you have a
mental illness. Get help, listen to your doctor and get on with it.
Seek all the help you can.

Acceptance is the willingness to stop the internal fight. It
brings great wisdom. I knew I was unwell after my Jesus Christ
episode at Broadmeadow in 2000, but I think it wasn't until after
the Anzac Day 2007 car crash that I was really shaken up enough
to become completely 100 per cent serious about my predicament. That was *seven years* of denial. I became psychotic again
straight after that and I remember telling myself: this is real. In
hindsight, I was dragged towards it kicking and screaming. Everyone around me accepted it quicker than I did: Louise, my mates;
they were straight on it. I was worried about being a burden, that
I might lose everyone if I became too hard to handle. 'Blokedom'
was part of it too—admitting to mental illness felt like weakness,
but the real weakness was in hiding my condition.

I now accept that I have a permanent, lifelong illness. So what?
Many other people have to accept serious illness which severely
impacts on their lives and the lives of their families. You can't
conquer bipolar; you can only manage it, and acceptance was the
first genuine step forward.

There are always going to be difficult days. It's always going to be a process. No-one is ever going to check out of hospital and be fine with it straight away: 'I've got bipolar, no worries. What are we having for lunch?' But the earlier the acceptance, the better. Mine has taken too long, but at least it's come. Day-to-day life has become easier. Mental illness doesn't make me a bad person. It doesn't make me inferior to anyone. Acceptance has made me comfortable about who I am. If you don't like it, no worries. I think there's a lot to like, which wasn't the case before I had bipolar. I don't lose sleep over it. I don't struggle to comprehend how my life took a sudden left turn. It is what it is. I have taken Louise's advice: I accept it's my responsibility. How I view the world and myself is up to me and no-one else. Mistakes are my own and I am responsible for my own happiness. The pursuit of perfection is guaranteed disappointment: perceived failure, regret, depression, loss of self-love and worse. I am what I am. I accept that belatedly but wholeheartedly, and I'm all the better for it.

2. Hope—and then make it happen

Few things are more valuable than hope. I have clung to it for dear sweet life. It was all I had in the darkest days and when I return to hardship, I'll reach for it again. Even if it doesn't feel like it, when you're in the deepest, darkest, ugliest, demon-filled hole of your life, hope will still be there. When you can't see it, trust it is there somewhere. Hope is from the heart. Anything in your heart is real.

> Hope gets me out of bed in the morning. Hope takes me to yoga classes. Hope ensures I will always take my medication.

Fear comes from your head. Your heart knows only hope. There is hope in any scenario, any predicament. It's a bigger lifeline than Lifeline. Think of your ideal outcome, even just one small sliver of a reason to keep going, and cling to that with all your might. In your best life, X would happen. Hang in there long enough to do X again, and celebrate it when you do.

Hope gets me out of bed in the morning. Hope takes me to yoga classes. Hope ensures I will always take my medication. I hope for a better life and then make it happen. I will keep hoping all the way through till my last breath. Why wouldn't I? Why wouldn't anyone? Hope for great things. I hate seeing people who are down and out. I can understand how they get there because I've been there myself. But it has to be fleeting. The saddest sight of all is someone who's given up.

One of my great lessons in hope came from a Victor E. Frankl's book, *Man's Search for Meaning*. Victor was a survivor of the Holocaust in a Nazi concentration camp. He never stopped looking for meaning and hope in the most desolate possible situation. He kept finding reasons to live. What Viktor Frankl went through makes me realise I've got it very good.

I tend to get a bit gung-ho when I read books like this, much to Louise's annoyance. I'll run up to her: 'Louise! You have to read this! I've learned some more, you won't believe it, you're going to love it!' She'll say, 'Craig, listen to me. I like reading fiction. How about I stick to the books I like, and you can read the ones you like.'

Louise keeps me grounded when I'm at risk of getting carried away. She tells me the things I need to hear—right before I go back to *Man's Search for Meaning*.

Trust in hope. Seek it. Acknowledge it. 'Faith is taking the first step when you can't see the top of the stairs,' said Martin Luther King Jnr. There are stages when that feels impossible. Which is why hope is valuable. The only replacement for lost hope is renewed hope.

I've had periods when I've thought I just cannot take one more second of this life. But each time, hope gets me through. It builds my levels of resilience. The next depression, I'm tougher than I was before. I have the proof I can survive. To use a football analogy, by the time you've played a hundred games, when you've been bashed around a bit for all those years, you're a better and braver player than you were before.

Another saying: 'If I think I can achieve something, I'm right. If I think I can't, I'm still right.' I'll never underestimate the power of my own thoughts.

3. Patience

I was impatient in every area of my life before diagnosis. I've learned patience. It's been a difficult lesson, but if I can change, you can. It depends how much we want it. I was an immediate-gratification person who had to slow down. I never savoured anything. It really was, 'What's next?' all the time. I believe in keeping busy and moving forward because I've also learned there's something to be said for timing.

> Peaks must have valleys. Life cannot be one long peak.

Charge forward at the right moments but take the foot off the accelerator when you can. Peaks must have valleys. Life cannot be one long peak. It's impossible because it's at odds with our humanity. Take a family holiday. (We have one every three months: we book it in advance so we have it to look forward to, so we know a rest is coming.) Sleep in every now and again. Put your feet up. Do nothing. There's an art to doing nothing. You can still get to your destination with your pedal not all the way to the metal. Immediacy isn't always ideal. I understand the rush that comes from quick fixes but there's also joy in the measured pursuit. I used to click my fingers and try and get what I wanted. If not, I would blow up. An hour later I'd frantically be looking for something else because the thrill of the previous chase was already over. Drag the chase out. Let it linger. Otherwise you've found a sure-fire way to blow a gasket.

Impatience is like perfectionism: a recipe for frustration, disappointment and anger. If you want and expect everything in your life to be perfect, right now, without so so much as a speck of dust, you're setting yourself up for a manic explosion or depression. The world has lots of dust. Do more than get used to it, embrace it! Get your hands dirty. It would be boring otherwise.

Patience is underrated. It's grateful and dignified.

My search for patience is not just inward. I want greater patience with other people. I want to expect less of them. I want to give them more time to come through if I'm waiting on them. I used to demand everything right away or there'd be hell to pay, but it feels good to be relaxing my demands. Patience is underrated. It's grateful and dignified.

I want to be mature enough to observe a situation before racing into judgement. I want to react wisely instead of over-emotionally. The better I become at this, the less stress I feel. I'm evolving and growing and I like it. Another pearl of wisdom: 'Only the very wise, and the very stupid, never change.' I'm constantly reminding myself to *breathe*. I think we take breathing for granted. There's nothing more important to us and nothing we think about less. Three slow, deep breaths immediately calm my mind. They remind me of the gift of being able to take them at all. The slower and more patient, the better.

4. Habits

I have habits I want and need to kick. I get frustrated when I fall back into a pattern of behaviour I thought I'd left behind. Those behaviours must be more deeply ingrained than I gave them credit for. There's a level of acceptance in this, too: only when I acknowledge them can I deal with them properly. I want to polish the parts of my behaviour still rough around the edges. If I only master one thing in my life, I want to make that one thing myself.

> I want to polish the parts of my behaviour still rough around the edges.

For example, I don't want to talk about myself so much. It must drive people nuts. Elka Graham, the Olympic swimming champion, has a great term for people who talk about themselves too much. She calls them 'optometrists': all they're worried about is the 'I's. I this, I that, I think . . . not a bad line. My goal is to shut up long enough to hear more about other people. A great Warren Ryan line is: 'There are two types of listeners. One who genuinely wants to hear what you've got to say and the other who just wants to know when to start talking again.' Communication is supposed to be a two-way street, not a dead end. It revolves around listening instead of talking. Every single person on this planet has a life story.

I want to be less loud in conversation. It drives me up the wall when I hear other people bellowing. 'Everything that irritates us about others can lead us to a better understanding of ourselves,' Carl Jung said. I want to listen more carefully. I want to be more present in a conversation instead of drifting away. I don't want to be nodding at a friend to give the impression of listening when I'm really only thinking about what I'm going to do after work, what's happening for dinner, what the footy score is. These are my issues and I'll do my best to not let them control my life. I will beat them, and I'll be a better person in umpteen regards when I do.

It's still a work in progress. I still occasionally revert to my old selfish ways. (I'm not hearing a word you're saying. I'm talking over the top of you. I don't want to see your point of view. You're wrong!) But it's becoming less frequent. The light bulb goes off: you're doing it again, stop being such a know-it-all, and snap out of it.

The results have been fantastic since I've flipped my old look-at-me-and-listen approach on its head. Don't underestimate the power to change the person you are. You can make minor modifications or have a complete overhaul. Don't overestimate your power to change others, either. They'll develop good habits by appreciating and mimicking yours. Cease worrying. Makes sense, doesn't it? What good does the worry do? Worrying is just another bad habit. So is chasing perfection. I learned a hard lesson there.

5. Discipline

I want the discipline required to take care of my mind, body and soul. Excessive use of alcohol, cigarettes and other illicit drugs are harmful and so I choose to go nowhere near them. They're all misguided forms of self-medication to deal with stress, anxiety and depression. And they are only delaying the inevitable. They do not do me one ounce of good, so they're out. There are no grey areas when it comes to discipline.

I want to be fit, and to be fit I need the discipline to do my weekly walk and other exercise routines. Exercise is nature's way of increasing the serotonin (the feel-good hormone) levels in the brain. Our bodies are designed to move, not sit still. The more exercise, the better I feel mentally as well as physically.

I want the discipline to keep up my medication routines and I want to be disciplined with my alternative therapies.

I want to do the things that make me smile.

Diet is crucial to my long-term health, so I want the discipline to keep junk food to the bare minimum. I think of my body as a mass of energy that will deplete and become listless and fatigued if I'm not aware of its needs. Your energy sources are like reserves of gold. Yoga helps to make me feel connected to whatever other forces might be at play around us. When mind, body and soul are in balance, you're smiling. That's the best possible outcome.

I want to do the things that make me smile. No self-discipline means not much hope. At best, life will become a shambles. At worst, a disaster. Routines are crucial to discipline. I want to be reliable, all the time. If I say I am going to meet you, I will be there.

If I get slack with one area of my life, it can spread like wildfire to others. One minute I'll be unfazed by being half-an-hour late for a meeting. My universe is affected because even if I pretend it's no big deal, my core knows it is. My universe has been thrown out of whack. Next, I'll get slack with something else. This attitude encourages shortcuts to be taken.

I think of my body as a mass of energy which will deplete and become listless and fatigued if I'm not aware of its needs.

At the other end of the scale, something small and seemingly insignificant as putting the litter in the bin plants a seed. Feels good. Feels *right*. Next thing, using the same discipline I'm starting to enjoy, I'm finishing every single task at work. Big things or small, the principles are the same. No matter what the situation, I want the discipline to do it right. Why? Because it's more fulfilling than half-baked alternatives.

6. Support and encouragement

It's an age-old requirement. 'Never discourage anyone who continually makes progress, no matter how slow,' Plato said. He could have stopped after the first three words. Never discourage anyone, ever, progress or not.

Encouragement can rear its beautiful head from anywhere. You don't need to be someone's best mate to help them out. A quick email, phone call or text can do the trick.

When Wayne Bennett was coaching St George Illawarra, he sent me an email one day when I was severely depressed and off work: 'Why weren't you on the radio today?' I replied that I was off work with depression. He responded: 'I thought that might have been the case. You should be a footy coach: we have that many highs and lows, we don't know if we're happy or depressed.' It gave me a laugh when I needed one. It was his way of showing support.

Humour can help any situation. Life is tough enough without focusing on the negatives. Who can help you see past them? Friends. Experts. Anyone you choose, and anyone who chooses to support and encourage you. In the toughest times of my life, when the seas have become especially stormy, that's when I've needed my support network. I'm blessed to have them and, when I'm well, I want to support and encourage them in return.

If you have a support crew to help you through, you're already halfway home. If not, I'd really encourage you to seek out organisations such as *beyondblue* or Lifeline. They will understand. It's what they're here for. At the very least, they'll be an outlet for you to express what you're going through. Just knowing someone is prepared to listen can be of enormous benefit, even down a telephone line to a stranger with a caring voice. Those who've grown up in less than ideal circumstances, who've had a really tough time when they're younger, can be tough cookies with strong survival techniques by the time they're in their mid-20s or mid-30s. Maybe we don't know how tough we are until we have to prove it. If you're doing this alone, I admire you immensely, but never be too proud to seek assistance. Support and encouragement can only help. Never be too shy to ask for a helping hand.

7. Honesty

I encourage us all to come clean about mental illness. An enormous burden was released when I stopped pretending. Honesty comes highly recommended. Most of us aspire to it, but I don't know if anyone has ever been 100 per cent honest 100 per cent of the time. I find it hard to imagine because I'm nowhere near it myself. Yet.

Don't we all tell little fibs to keep the peace sometimes? What I've learned, however, is that the more things in life I'm upfront and honest about, the lighter my load is. Just telling the truth does make a difference. With everything. It's fantastically liberating. You've got nothing to fear because nothing is being hidden.

Being honest has an actual physical effect on me. I get lighter on my feet when I've owned up to something that's been bugging me. It's hard to say the words, but it's such a relief afterwards. Invariably, coming clean isn't half as hard as we think it's going to be. I might be dreading saying it but then it comes out and . . . it's OK! I haven't been struck down by lightning, the seas haven't parted. As the reaction to Andrew Johns's and Wally Lewis's disclosures shows, people actually think more of you. Even better, you think more of yourself. The truth really does set you free!

We all have things in our life that not everyone knows about—that's human nature. I think everyone has at least one little secret they will take to their grave. It's private and that's fine by me. There are parts of all our lives we don't feel obligated to share, but when it comes to mental illness, it cannot be put in a secret drawer. Honesty is the next step from acceptance. I don't feel frightened of telling people about my condition. I'd be more uneasy if I was involved in a cover up. *That* is what would keep me up at night. (Who knows? When so-and-so said such-and-such, was that a hint that they know?)

> Being honest has an actual physical effect on
> me. I get lighter on my feet when I've owned up to
> something that's been bugging me.

My bipolar has been known for a while now: even at the very start there were witnesses to events at the train station. I couldn't tell those people fast enough! I wanted them to know there was a proper medical cause for what happened. I just think, what's the point in denial? Honesty is a blessing, blatantly and in disguise.

8. Self-respect

I want to feel comfortable in my own skin. I think that would be the greatest gift: if I could guarantee my kids have one trait, it might just be this. It's taken me more than 40 years to feel as if I'm getting there. Don't you wait that long! I have just reached a point where I'm relaxed and realise that this is me, and I don't mind it one bit! Australian men can shy away from those kind of thoughts because self-respect gets confused with self-absorption. No-one likes a smart arse. We're all to scared of being regarded as one so we go too far the other way.

Being comfortable with yourself doesn't mean you get arrogant or dismissive. It doesn't make you superior to anyone else. On the contrary, it makes you comfortable enough to be in the company of anyone. It's about having your own standards, your own set of values and being prepared to live by them. It's not a stretch. You *want* to live by them because you know they're right. It's so right it's nearly comical. They're what works for you. Self-respect, in the really big picture, is being satisfied when I go to bed at night that I'm happy with everything I've done that day. Well, maybe not *happy*—but everything I've done that day I can live with. I can live with myself and my decisions and how they've impacted on other people. I sleep well because my conscience is clear.

My medication helps, but a clear, satisfied conscience can be the most uplifting yet calming force there is. A lack of self-respect can be paralysing and destructive. I've come to realise my conscience can't be lied to. That's not to say I haven't made mistakes during the course of a day. I don't expect that of myself. There will always be things I regret or think I could have done better. But I like the feeling of knowing the motives for my actions and words have been positive.

There's a daily review: could I have done anything better? Should I have said that? Next time, I will. Patience is a must here, too. The beauty is that it's win–win. If it's all gone well during the day, that's great. If not, at least I've learned something. The next day is a fresh start, another chance to put my ideals into practice. I try to build on that, day by day, more and more bricks, until there's a very strong foundation.

Self-respect is looking at yourself and liking what you see. It's not about physical appearance, it's about who you are and what you stand for. Being comfortable with what you see and think. It doesn't matter who you are or what you're doing, at the end of the day, every single person in this world has to go to sleep with their own thoughts. Whether you're a murderer or a saint, we all have to put our heads down at night and think about what we've done.

I used to need company all the time. I don't any more. I like having a bit of time to myself. I can sit in the sun for an hour with a cup of tea, happy as can be. That's a fantastic breakthrough. I can put my feet up and do a Sudoku puzzle and be blissfully happy. I love the feeling of doing nothing when the time is right, just consciously doing nothing except relaxing.

Giving myself enough sleep: that's self-respect.

Did my diagnosis harm my self-respect? No. Oddly enough, it was the first step towards gaining it because it made me confront myself. In a lot of ways, it probably brought to a head the traits I wasn't entirely impressed with. The diagnosis was the *start* of self-respect. That is the least likely outcome I would have predicted that day at Broadmeadow. It changed the direction of my life, another good thing because it sent me in another direction. I'm a better person for it. I was on a path to self-destruction, and I did destruct.

Everyone needs self-respect to treat themselves well. Eating well: that's self-respect. Giving myself enough sleep: that's self-respect. Now there's just knowledge, the sense of everything being more than OK. Whatever's in my past it doesn't matter because that's exactly what it is: the past. I have to settle everything down or I know the repercussions. I get rewards from doing the right things. That seems a very fair deal to me.

I have finally worked out that you can't be all things to all people. I've simply stopped trying to be. Bliss! Problem solved! It doesn't matter what anyone else thinks about you. It's what you think about you that's important. Who is directing your life? Who is making the important decisions? Who is in control? Who is responsible? If the answer isn't 'I am' every time, it might be an idea to look closely at who is. And then do something about it.

9. Resilience

I've been thinking about an old saying: 'What doesn't kill you, makes you stronger.' Here's my take: it's only true if you learn your lesson from the experience. If you get hit by a car while crossing the road without looking both ways and you survive, there's no guarantee you'll survive a second time if you repeat your mistake. Every time we stuff up, there's a lesson to be learned. My worst day? It's difficult to nail it down to one in particular—there've been a few rough ones! But I would say the worst was when I tried to shake off a million cobwebs of depression by going for a run. I ended up in front of the local church. I just broke down and prayed. That's a day that will forever be in my memory because I think that was the lowest of all the lows. I was suicidal and just a mess. The church is just around the corner from where we still live, so there's a constant reminder to look after myself otherwise I might end up weeping at the church doors again. Prayer is underrated. Having been through all that, I'm able to appreciate the umpteen fantastic days that have followed.

I've had far more good days than bad with bipolar. It's a blessing to be able to say that. And all the more reason to be grateful that I could tough it out when I had to. As Thomas Edison said: 'Many of life's failures are people who did not realise how close they were to success when they gave up.' My good days, when the heart sings and I feel good about myself and the world around me, when I'm treating people exactly how I want to, easily outweigh the bad days. They're treasured because I know the other side. How people treat me in return is immaterial: I just want to treat them well. I think one follows the other anyway. The world and its inhabitants don't owe me a thing. Resilience has stopped me from capitulating. I refuse to. Life is too precious.

I need resilience to ignore the temptation of the high. It's my overriding ambition: to keep the mania away. Plus-two and plus-three are absolutely no-go zones and it takes strength to ignore them. The temptation is to tiptoe in, have a bit of fun and get out before it's too late. But plus-three is Hotel California: I'm not allowed to leave. An experiment to try for those of you who, like me, have a mind that sometimes goes into overdrive and is prone to mania. I have discovered the puzzle game Sudoku in the past year and believe it or not it seems to be helping me to stay on the straight and narrow. I reckon it might have something to do with the right and left hemispheres in our brain. This is just my theory but consider this. Creativity is said to be a right-brain thing, logic and rational thinking a left-brain function. I have always been very poor at mathematics. I just didn't get it and still don't. My strengths have always been communicating, writing and so on. So I believe Sudoku forces me to use the left side of my brain. When I started Sudoku puzzles I was hopeless but I have become progressively better at them. Still not great but better. Maybe even this simple exercise has helped re-balance my brain. I don't know; it's just a theory, but I think it has helped to ground me when I sometimes tend to fly off creatively. Give it a go.

When depression comes knocking on my door again, which I know it will, I'll be more resilient than ever: I've got enough memories of the good times to know it's worth coming out the other side. Louise and I are going to have a big overseas trip one day. The kids are at a fascinating stage, moving through their teens and into adulthood. There has been sadness and happiness because of my condition but I am resilient enough to get through. There may be the black dog and sunshine. There will always be light and shade. All those will pass. They're all part of what is making this a very full life. I will face adversity again. The only thing that matters will be my response. I am up for the fight.

10. Faith

I have an increasingly persistent feeling that it's important. Life is a smoother ride when I'm feeling strong in my faith. Is it a faith in God? It's a faith in something much bigger than me, bigger than all of us, and very difficult to comprehend. Investigations are set to continue. I've really struggled with faith at certain stages in my life. At the worst times of my life, I've thought about the poem 'Footprints in the Sand'. The narrator of the poem is looking back at his life as two sets of footprints along the sand on a beach. The two sets of footprints are his own, and God's. At the most harrowing points of his life, he sees just one set of prints. The narrator asks God why, in the toughest parts of my life, when I really needed you, did you abandon me? God replies: there's only one set of footprints because at those times, I was carrying you.

I relate to that poem very much. It's one of many written works that really made me contemplate a bigger picture. Little kids ask 'Why?' all the time. 'It's bedtime', 'Why?', 'Because you need to sleep', 'Why?' In adulthood I'm still asking 'Why?': We are here. Why? Why? Why? I just really want to know! How I came to read 'Footprints in the Sand' still amazes me. I could have so easily never seen it at all.

I was at the Merewether Golf Club in Newcastle, in the main bar area, when a man, whom I had never met, just walked up out of nowhere and gave it to me. He was aware of my bipolar. He just walked up and said: 'Here, take this with you' as he handed over a piece of paper. I read it there and then, and I've never forgotten it. That man has no idea what he did for me that day. I'd never seen him before, and I've never seen him again. What a

fantastically wonderful thing for him to have done. He gave me
a great gift with that poem, but wanted nothing in return.

> When I'm living in faith that everything will be fine,
> I really do think I'm living life *right.*

Everything I have come to think about faith is encapsulated
in the words he gave me: another step on the spiritual journey
I've talked about. When I'm living in faith that everything will
be fine, I really do think I'm living life *right.* It's a feeling that has
only increased since I started writing this book. A new part of me
is opening up: I like it so much I'm not going to place any limits
on it. In tough times, it has sustained me as though it's the most
powerful form of hope there is. In good times, I'm more humble
and appreciative of the gifts around me.

I remember about twenty years ago saying to a really good
mate of mine: 'Look, I don't know about this whole faith thing,
the whole God thing. I just really don't know if I believe *any*
of it. Sorry, I'm just being honest with you.' He looked at me
with understanding but said something that stuck in my memory
for all time: 'Mate, I don't know how you get through the day
without it.' At the time I had no idea what he meant but something about his reply, and the way he delivered it, stayed with me,
lodged itself in my brain.

Now I completely understand what he was saying. Life can
be tough if you don't have faith in something. I believe in
believing. I'm not telling anyone what they should believe
in, but it strikes me that people with belief do have a different
air about them. All their actions and words and thoughts serve
a higher purpose: it's the ultimate form of giving and, best of
all, helping.

Maybe it just comes from reaching a more mature age, when
I've really settled down into family life, lived a bit, been beaten

up a bit. You're always going to ask yourself different questions in your 40s and 50s than in your 20s and 30s. You start realising you're not going to be here forever: why have I been put here in the first place? The more you've lived, the more you have to look back on . . . what purpose has it all served? When you're younger, all you're doing is looking ahead, as you should.

I'm more than halfway through my life and there's been a seismic shift in outlook. All I know is this: well, I don't *know* anything, but I have an unshakable feeling that we're involved in a far bigger game than we're aware of. That this earthly world of ours is just part of something bigger. What it really entails, I have no idea! But I honestly think every single one of us is caught up in the same game. I like the thought of all of us being involved. I always go back to that poem. For me, every time it's necessary for me to be carried, it's as though all the people around me have been strategically put in place by a higher force to do the job. It's not one person, or one event, that gets us though.

People arrive in your world at precisely the moment when they can provide exactly what you need to keep going, or vice versa, and then we step out of each other's picture again. I think that's true for all of us—as if we've served the divine purpose we had in each other's lives. The man who gave me a copy of 'Footprints in the Sand' is the perfect case in point, fuelling my ever-skyrocketing belief there's a bigger game at play.

11. Live life

Today is the most important day of my life. Past mistakes: they don't matter. Today is the only day we have. Yesterday is gone. Tomorrow is yet to arrive. Today, today, today. It matters little how I began my life or what happened in the middle. The most important thing is how I finish the race. First impressions last? The last impressions carry more weight.

When Muhammad Ali was asked how he'd like to be remembered, he said: 'As someone who took a few cups of love, a tablespoon of patience, a teaspoon of generosity, a pint of kindness, a quart of laughter, a pinch of concern and then he mixed willingness with happiness, he added lots of faith and then he stirred it up well and then he spread it over the span of a lifetime and served it to each and every deserving person he met.' I love that. That's how I want to live.

My attitude will shape my world. I *will* be happy. I will suck the marrow out of every year I have left. Can my bipolar pass? Can it be cured? According to modern medicine and Dr Weiss, no. I'm OK with that. It's my lifetime companion, this stranger inside me, and I accept that now. For a long time I didn't and I was determined to beat it, only to end up back in hospital. Now I beat it by controlling it as best I can. It can be a pain in the neck but I'm used to having it around.

If bipolar make its presence felt again, I will accept that, but I refuse to fret over where and when. I've gone nearly two years now without trouble. That's a win. I've written this book. All I can do from here is look after myself; listen to my doctor, who has been a wonderful influence; listen to Louise; have faith that our best years are still to come. It is impossible for me to do any more. I pray when it gets tough and feel thankful when it's not. I refuse to live in fear because fear is the opposite of faith.

My greatest strength is the trust I have that I can and will get through whatever is thrown at me. There are going to be more trials and tribulations. There will be more depressions and flights of crazy ideas. So what? That's life for every one of us, even if we experience these things on different scales. It's all part of our varying degrees of the same human condition.

> My greatest strength is the trust I have that I can and will get through whatever is thrown at me.

Who I really am will be determined by my responses. I want mine to be inspired by dignity and grace, but I have no interest in being perfect. The more imperfect, the better. It's human. I'm going to revel in my imperfection. Who knows, maybe I'll completely fall off the road. Life is what happens when you're busy making other plans, as Lennon sang, but at least I know where the road is now. It's a wonderful thing to have had these experiences and survived them.

There's a great line in the movie *Braveheart*. It gives me a chill every time I hear it, say it or think of it, which is a lot. William Wallace is addressing the clans before leading the Scots into battle against the English. His men are reluctant to fight because they're hopelessly outnumbered and fear they're about to be slaughtered. 'Every man dies,' says William Wallace. 'But not every man truly lives.' If I embrace that as a mantra, through good times and bad, I can never go too far wrong. I am going to die one of these days. To know that is a blessing. It rids me of complacency.

What happens between now and my last day is entirely up to me. That's a powerful thought. Am I OK, mate? Yes. Life is for living. Believe me, it can all change in a split second but through ridiculous highs and dungeon-lows, count me in. There have been many people who have helped me, inspired me, educated me and just been there when I have needed them throughout this journey. Just by being a friend, an acquaintance or someone who has made contact by email or letter they have had an impact on my life. This doesn't even begin to measure the support and impact of my family over the years. The love and support of my parents, Dick and Maureen, my brother Ian and sister Kate have made a huge difference to me. Many family members can and do walk away when confronted with a serious mental illness. My family haven't.

In closing, consider all the things that wear you down, make you tired, stress you out. The things making you anxious, depressed and angry. Write them on a piece of paper. As you (and no-one else) is in charge of your life, make a conscious decision to get rid of them. Try it.

Consider all the things that energise and inspire you. The things that engage you. The things providing laughter and relaxation. The sources of peace and calm in your world. Write them on a piece of paper. As you (and no-one else) is in charge of your life, make a conscious decision to embrace them like never before. Go on, try it.

Afterword from a friend

Over the years since his breakdown on the eve of the Sydney Olympics and subsequent diagnosis with bipolar, Craig has faced an ongoing challenge to find balance that enables him to manage his illness. This quest hasn't been easy nor always achievable, evidenced by some periods of hospitalisation. I am reminded of Craig's ongoing battle through the words of 'These Days' by Powderfinger. The shadow cast, the darkness of the troughs, creeping into his life, are the realities of not finding the right balance. If *Broken Open* was the tale of one man's journey back from the brink of hell, then *A Better Life* is the tale of that same man's ongoing challenge to manage his life and also his commitment to raise awareness and to help others.

I have known Craig for literally longer than I can remember. We began our school days together. The year was 1968 and the first vivid memory I have from those days is playing the game 'Red Rover', a 'tough' tackle game that helped prepare us for Rugby Union in later years. Right through school we were great mates. This friendship is just as strong today. We always had a fierce but friendly rivalry when it came to all sporting contests, albeit in the slightly more sedate surroundings of the golf course these days. We completed our secondary education at Singleton High where I can't help but think both of us would have achieved better results if sport had been a HSC subject in those days.

Craig has been fortunate to be able to roll his passion for sport into his daily work. Away from his radio work, he has dedicated much of his time to raising awareness of mental health issues.

I recently came across a quote attributed to rugby league coach Wayne Bennett in which he said: 'The highest reward for a person's toil is not what they get for it but what they become by it.' Craig has endured some tough periods and I sense that from this he has emerged a better person, one who shows more compassion and empathy than he previously may have.

Life may not have turned out as Craig had planned but, far from letting it slip through his hands, he has grasped it and embraced new challenges. This has not only made his life better but also the lives of the people he meets. He is making a difference and for this he can be proud.

I hope you have enjoyed reading Craig's thoughts, that they give answers for some of you and raise questions for others. I'll leave you with the words of Canadian author Robin Sharma, which I came across in Justin Langer's book *Seeing the Sunrise*. I feel they are an appropriate summation of Craig's journey this past while.

Our wounds ultimately give us wisdom.
Our stumbling blocks inevitably become our stepping stones.
And our setbacks lead us to our strengths.

Barry Smith

Top shelf: the books that have changed me

As well as all of the people who have come along for the ride, there have been some wonderful books that have been great companions and sources of learning. There are many more, but I have narrowed this list down to my favourite fifteen.

Albom, Mitch *Tuesday's with Morrie: An old man, a young man and life's greatest lessons*, Broadway Books, New York, 2002.

Coelho, Paulo *Manual of the Warrior Light*, HarperCollins, New York, 1997.

Coelho, Paulo *The Alchemist*, HarperCollins, New York, 2006.

Dalai Lama, His Holiness the *The Art of Happiness: A handbook for living*, Riverhead Books, New York, 1998.

Demartini, John *The Gratitude Effect: The inner power series*, Burman Books, Scarborough Canada, 2007.

Frankl, Victor E. *Man's Search for Meaning: An introduction to logotherapy*, Beacon Press, Boston MA, 2006.

Gibran, Kahlil *The Prophet*, Alfred A. Knopf, New York, 1995.

Moore, Thomas *Dark Nights of the Soul: A guide to finding your way through life's ordeals*, Gotham, New York, 2005.

Myss, Caroline *Anatomy of the Spirit: The seven stages of power and healing*, Three Rivers Press, New York, 1997.

Tolle, Eckhart *The Power of Now: A guide to spiritual enlightenment*, New World Library, Novato CA, 2004.

Yancey, Philip *Soul Survivor: How thirteen unlikely mentors helped my faith survive the church*, WaterBrook Press, Colorado Springs, 2003.

Yancey, Philip *Prayer: Does it make any difference?*, Zondervan, Grand Rapids MI, 2006.

Yogananda, Paramahansa *How to be Happy All the Time: The wisdom of Yogananda*, Crystal Clarity Publishers, California, 2006.

Yogananda, Paramahansa *Autobiography of a Yogi*, Empire Books, Greensboro NC, 2011.

Zukav, Gary *The Seat of the Soul*, Free Press, Hemel Hempstead, 1990.